Meats & Sweets
A High Vitality Diet

Tracy A. Minton-Matesz
&
Don A. Matesz

Meats & Sweets
A High Vitality Diet

by Tracy A. Minton-Matesz
&
Don Matesz

Please note that this is intended as educational in nature, not as a substitute for the advice of your physician. Please consult your primary health care practitioner when making any big changes to your diet, and do your own research as necessary and appropriate. Your health is your responsibility.

MEATS & SWEETS
A High Vitality Diet

First Edition

Copyright © 2019 by
Tracy A. Minton-Matesz & Donald A. Matesz
All rights reserved. No part of this book may be reproduced, scanned, or distributed in any printed or electronic form without permission. Any information used must be attributed to the source.

First Edition: November 2019
Printed in the United States of America

ISBN: 9781701925021

Cover photo:
Scrambled eggs with cheese, turkey sausage, & fruit lovingly prepared by the staff at Le Peep, Evanston
Photo copyright of Tracy Minton-Matesz

1 - INTRODUCTION 9

Our Journey to Meats & Sweets 16

We Need More Than High Vitality Foods To Thrive.... 23

2 - WHY A HIGH VITALITY DIET? 29

What Foods Best Support Human Nature? 29

Why We Need Meats 44

Benefits of Milk & Calcium 50

Moderating Meat Intake 57

Gelatin 64

The Sweets ~ Fruits and Honey 68

What About Grains? 73

What About Vegetables? 75

3 - THE 3 TIERS OF FOODS 87

Tier 1 Foods 89

Tier 2 Foods 90

Tier 3 Foods 92

Food Selection Guidelines 93

What About Weight Loss? 96

Trouble Shooting 104

4 - MEATS 111

Eggs 111

Beef, Fish, Poultry & Pork 116

Slow Roasting Method 135

Bone Broth & Soups 146

5 - SWEETS 153

Fruit Salads 153

Jello Recipes 160

More Sweet Treats 168

6 - CARROT SALADS 174

7 - VEGGIE SIDES 177

8 - BEVERAGES 182

6 - RESOURCES 187

1 - INTRODUCTION

MEATS & SWEETS ~ A HIGH VITALITY DIET emphasizes foods which will rev up (versus slow down) your metabolism, increase energy, and support the health of your endocrine system (especially your thyroid gland), and digestive system ~ both central to shielding against the negative effects of stress. Stress is a major factor undermining health which too few diet gurus and 'authorities' are discussing.

MEATS & SWEETS is *not* a restrictive, authoritarian approach telling you what to eat, and what to avoid. Instead, foods are prioritized in tiers to help you make the best choices for *your* particular geographical location, and personal needs. Our desire is to provide clear information, especially for those who want to *optimize their genetic potential* for a healthy, sweet life!

MEATS & SWEETS is a major paradigm shift with respect to how you think about health. We encourage consumption of foods many now avoid. We also encourage you to learn to trust your instincts, or as we often say, *your true nature*, as a more empowering system of finding *your own personal sweet spot*, while enjoying a high vitality life!

Don and I believe it is well past time to abandon one-size-fits-all approaches which typically dictate restriction or avoidance of one or the other macronutrients, i.e. carbohydrate, protein, or fat ~ or entire food groups such as all animal or plant foods ~ as a means of achieving fast weight loss.

Instead, we recommend making the optimal and healthy functioning of *all* of your physiological systems as *your top priority* for a high vitality life. Rather than focus on the numbers on the scale, turn more inwards, and sense the subtle changes that will begin to occur when you eat the right foods, and support your diet as needed with appropriate supplementation.

While many of the popular trending diets including vegan, raw, ketogenic, low-carb or zero carb/carnivore may provide benefits ~ at least initially ~ the question remains, are they actually sustainable *long-term*? Can these diets which exclude either all or most animal *or* plant foods provide the nutrition required to achieve **optimal** vitality and health for the long haul? As you will see in Chapter 2, too little *and* too much of both the meats (protein and fat) and sweets (primarily fruit and honey) can bring about many health imbalances that are cumulative over time.

Can you achieve safe, healthy (versus *fast*) weight loss, **increase** your energy, eliminate cravings, and feel your best ~ physically and mentally ~ by eating in a manner that is simple, enjoyable, and sustainable *for life*? Without feeling restricted? We believe you can ~ but first, let's define what we mean by *health*.

By whole health, we mean the following:

- Your endocrine system is functioning well, which involves several glands including the pituitary, thyroid, adrenal glands, liver, and reproductive glands. Ideally, these glands communicate harmoniously to produce hormones which are fundamental to homeostatic balance and health, including metabolism, ability to tolerate cold or heat, sweating, appetite, blood sugar balance, moods, sex drive, sleep, fertility, and much more. As an example, depression, anxiety, chronically cold hands and feet, and weight gain that is difficult to lose are a few symptoms that indicate hypothyroid function. I list more symptoms of thyroid imbalances in Chapter 3.
- Ability to achieve & maintain your ideal percent body fat and weight.
- A well functioning digestive system: ability to consume a variety of healthy foods, extract the energy, assimilate nutrients, and consistent, regular elimination of healthy formed log-shaped, easy to pass stools with minimal odor.
- Lustrous skin, strong nails, and healthy hair, without excess hair loss.

- Stress, worry, anxiety, and depression are minimal or well managed. Stress truly can be a 'hidden killer' if not understood and managed through proper diet and lifestyle practices.
- Personally appropriate mental clarity and cognitive functioning, and physical vitality.
- Free of unhealthful cravings and addictions.
- Sound sleep through the night, waking refreshed.
- Relatively free of pain, or abnormal swelling, inflammation, or other symptoms impeding productivity and enjoyment of your life.
- Blood tests reveal *optimal* ranges of required nutrients, hormones, etc.

Additionally, having a positive mental attitude is difficult to achieve when the brain is malnourished. Contrarily, a positive mindset can help one to transcend many health and life challenges! Most of us are not symptom-free, but we can do our best to *optimize our potential*, and *minimize* genetic expression of disease, *and* dis-ease.

Don't you finally want to find a way to eat that is healthy, balanced, simple, enjoyable, flexible, *and* doesn't entail having to forever forgo some of your favorite foods, or even an entire category of foods, whether all plants, meats, dairy, fruits or healthy sweets? Think long-term satisfaction, and graceful aging versus short-term, instant gratification that may not be sustainable. High vitality living in *your* sweet spot, versus constant avoidance and restriction.

Well get ready for this one. You may want to sit down, and grab a spoon! With our **MEATS & SWEETS** approach, you now have permission to eat ice cream! And even a little cheesecake here and there!

Okay, before everyone lets out a resounding, "Yipee!" or "You're nuts!", in chapter two Don explains *why* a **MEATS & SWEETS** approach provides the *right blend* of nutrients to help you best thrive. In a nutshell, *meats* including a variety of meats, organs, eggs, dairy and shellfish, and *sweets* ~ primarily from fresh and/or dried fruits, juices, honey, and possibly tree saps ~ are complementary foods that **best** optimize metabolic efficiency, hormonal balance, and your ability to minimize the negative effects of stress, and maximize wellbeing.

Yes, milk, eggs, and sugar (including ice cream) can be included on your menu ~ providing you choose the right kind with the fewest ingredients, (such as several Håagen Dazs flavors) ~ or better, learn to make your own! Likewise, *sometimes* a little cheesecake and a latte or steamed milk can be the perfect snack! It's my go-to choice while traveling, especially at certain airports (like Ely's Cheesecake at Chicago O'Hare!)

Because *meats* and *sweets* have both been increasingly vilified in main stream outlets, and many are confused about whether to be high or low protein, fat, or carb, Chapter 2, *What Is A High Vitality Diet?* is intended to be *just enough* information ~ without getting too bogged down ~ explaining *why* we consider **MEATS & SWEETS** to be a high vitality approach. For more in-depth research, look for Don's revised edition of **THE HYPERCARNIVORE DIET** in 2020. You may also want to read our free e-book, **10 RARELY DISCUSSED REASONS PEOPLE FAIL TO THRIVE ON** *ANY* **DIET** ~ available at Live-Fruitfully.com.

Truth is, people are quick to vilify many foods these days, parroting popular nutrition trends. For example, many now consider carrots to be 'worse than candy' yet this is based on the erroneous notion that carrots are high glycemic, without understanding glycemic load. The theory is that consumption of carrots (and likewise fruit) will spike blood sugar, yet this isn't the case. Rather, both are a great source of quick energy, and can be especially beneficial for between meal snacks. Let's look at how others view carrots.

In **THE CHEROKEE HERBAL**, by J.T. Garret, herbs and plants are considered according to the four directions, each with their own focus. Carrots were used in 'West Medicine' which "focused on the internal aspects of the physical body." According to Garret, "Carrot plants…were used as natural energy bars (especially for those with hypoglycemia), chronic diarrhea bouts, and as a "cleanser" for the intestinal tract. Carrot was included in tonic formulas and was cooked with other plants and fed to infants and children with diarrhea. Raw carrots are used today for developing strength of ballplayers and competitors. Carrots are high in pectin fiber."

According to **Chinese Dietary Therapy,** edited by Liu Jilin and Gordon Peck, "Carrot has a sweet flavor, a Neutral nature and a propensity for the Spleen, Liver and Lung channels. It has effects of reinforcing the Spleen, aiding digestion, reinforcing the Liver, promoting acuity of vision, sending down Counterflow Qi, arresting cough, clearing up Heat and detoxifying."

They list applications for using carrot as follows:

- For indigestion, stagnancy of food, fullness in the abdomen, or difficult stool, take cooked carrots with sugar. Its effect can be enhanced when taken with turnip as well.
- For blurred vision owing to deficiency in the Liver, night blindness, infantile malnutrition, dry eyes, take carrots cooked with lard, or in a soup cooked with pig's liver. (Pig's liver nourishes the yin.)
- For cough due to Lung Heat, take carrot juice on its own or make a decoction with Chinese dates.
- For fever and measles failing to erupt thoroughly in children, take carrots with water chestnuts and coriander.

This is an example of how every herb, plant, or food can be used as medicine, yet at the wrong time, or dose, it can become like a toxin. Our Western approach tends to reduce foods into isolated components, but there are many more ways to view foods, depending on one's perspective.

Our Journey to Meats & Sweets

In 2016, after over five years following a produce-rich, plant-based, macrobiotic diet emphasizing 'grains, greens, and beans', we eliminated *all* the grains and beans, and added in small portions of lean meats, and more fruit.

We made the change because we were having several 'failure to thrive' issues, which for me included: ongoing fatigue, difficulty getting going in the morning, low motivation, low libido, cold hands and feet, difficulty retaining information, ashen, dry skin, dry hair, seemingly accelerated wrinkling and graying, regular bouts of constipation despite a high-fiber, whole foods diet, lower belly bloating, blood sugar imbalances (with postural hypotensive episodes of feeling like I was about to drop, followed by mini seizure-like jerking sensations), ongoing stiffness, joint pain and tendonitis, sinus congestion and phlegm, lowered immune system, bad allergies, and more. Don was having horrible gas, psoriasis, injuries that were not healing, and towards the end, an insatiable craving for protein that finally drove us back to eating meat again after a five year abstinence. While we felt great when we initially began a plant-based diet, we found it increasingly difficult to sustain.

Upon switching out the grains and beans for eggs, fish, and lean meats, we immediately experienced an increase in our energy, and a profusion of circulation enhancing our skin. Don had less gas, and I felt my motivation and pep return. We pegged the way we were eating *Meats & Sweets* as the inclusion of more potassium-rich fruit ~ fresh, stewed, dried, and baked ~ seemed an ideal complement to more sodium-rich meats, however, we continued to consume nuts, seeds, and **lots** of dark leafy greens and vegetables, while avoiding dairy foods.

Within several months of adding meat back into our diet, we stumbled upon some intriguing information indicating that all those greens and vegetables we believed to be 'nature's pharmacy' contained oxalate acids and other troubling compounds that could impair gut and thyroid health, as Don explains in Chapter 2. There was a growing movement of people who were forgoing ALL plant foods, apparently with great results, not only with weight loss, but overcoming joint pain, auto-immune conditions, depression, and more. This was an entirely new angle we had *never* previously considered. Out of curiosity, we began to experiment with eliminating more plant foods, ultimately obtaining 90%+ of our total calories from animal foods. Our excess fat dropped off, body composition improved, and Don's psoriasis began to clear, *for the first time in over forty years!* It seemed like magic! Don wrote **The Hypercarnivore Diet** ~ a culmination of many years of research and direct experience. Hypercarnivore is the biological term for animals who derive 70% or greater total calories from consumption of animals. Don recommended a whole foods, animal-centered diet, prioritizing fruits above other plant foods, while encouraging readers to determine for themselves what they best tolerate.

As if on cue, after initially feeling great, progress stalled, again. The longer we continued a very low-carb diet, the more we experienced both new and old symptoms. The most disabling for Don was the cramping pain in his legs and feet waking him up several times a night, and in his abdomen while training.

We both had fat creep back on. I began to crave sweets, often not knowing what to eat to feel satisfied (because you know, sugar and fruit are off the menu in these circles, although I did still eat seasonal berries.)

Major drowsiness post meals unexpectedly returned, which I experienced on the higher-carb, plant-based diet. There were other symptoms as well. Don had periodic bouts of intense abdominal pain, causing the need to abstain from food for sometimes 48 hours; our nails were getting brittle again, and as you can imagine, successive nights of being woken by cramps, *and a lack of sugar* can lead to increased irritability.

I share our story because as it turns out, we are not alone. We have heard from several others who had been trying to follow Zero Carb/Carnivore or Ketogenic diets, and after some time, began to have similar symptoms.

More recently, Don began reading many articles written by biologist and researcher, Ray Peat, PhD. He followed Peat's trail of references, and did more of his own research, partly motivated by the desire to heal conditions that had yet to fully resolve no matter what our approach, especially what remained of his psoriasis. **MEATS & SWEETS, A HIGH VITALITY DIET** is thus inspired in part by the extensive work of Dr. Ray Peat, especially with helping shed light on the function of fructose, thyroid health, the damaging effects of stress, and much more.

Don and I have since connected the dots better than we had previously. Through our willingness to be open to new information, and discover for ourselves through direct experience, we have now learned more acutely what our upper and lower limits of carbohydrates, protein, and fats are, something we encourage you to discover for yourself as well.

Each of the the previously mentioned approaches to eating brought some relief ~ at least initially ~ yet predictably stalled, as other issues surfaced. Peat considers each of these approaches ~ the *eat this, not that* emphasis on macronutrient restrictions, i.e. low versus high-carb, protein, &/or fat, *or* the *exclusion* of either *all* animal foods (vegan diets), all plant foods (Zero Carb / Carnivore Diet), and others ~ to be more authoritarian in nature, only working for some people, some of the time. However, despite our personal disappointments over the years achieving results, then seeing the progress seemingly slip away, we gained valuable insights into the entire nutritional puzzle, some of which may have only been discovered because of our own health challenges, and dogged determination to not just heal, but to thrive.

Adding some carbohydrate back into our diet in the form of fruit, honey, and syrup immediately stopped Don's cramping. In early 2019, I had essentially lost the use of my right hand as my thumb had become nearly inoperable at the main and distal joints. I believed it to be a result of occupational overuse from reflexology and typing. After months of no sign of improvement, I began to wonder if I would have to have it operated on, however, I was not wanting to do so unless there was no other choice. The tendon at the main joint stuck out, and was visibly inflamed. The distal joint would lock up, requiring me to use my other hand to straighten it. Each time I bent or straightened my knuckle, it snapped. The thumb showed no signs of improvement for months while following a super low-carb diet. Immediately after adding fruit back into my diet, it began to heal. Within no time, the inflammation was gone, and I could again use my thumb, and regain the strength of my right grip.

I can also sense the ease to my nervous system when I up my fructose/sugar consumption while under stress. Others have also commented about how much better their mood is when they add a little carbohydrate back into their diet. Our sleep is better too. I do not have any blood sugar imbalance issues either. I did while eating a diet high in 'complex carbs' or starches, and I began to have issues after being on a super low carb, Keto-Carnivore diet for about one year.

Ultimately, our goal is to free ourselves from restrictive ideologies that limit our ability to experience a fruitful life. As an example, our experiences taught us that we don't have to eat tons of kale and greens in order to thrive. If hungry and away from home, we can make do quite simply by buying a half gallon of milk, and possibly some grapes or other fresh or dried fruit, then head to a park and get our fill on a fraction of what it would cost us to eat out, avoiding unwanted excess sodium or unhealthful PUFA oils commonly used in most restaurants ~ all while eating outdoors!

When making any dietary changes, it is not uncommon to experience a mix of positive improvements, and uncomfortable symptoms. This is normal. The key is to learn how to discern which symptoms are a sign of progress, and which are not.

Considering the bulk of people have some level of digestive dysfunction, among other potential health imbalances, the majority of seeming negative symptoms ~ bloating, gas, and changes to bowel health ~ may be the very symptoms that take a bit of time to resolve. Patience may be required to heal the gut, clear out endotoxins, and restore a healthy flora and balance. To repeat, this is a *trust your true nature* approach. That means we encourage you to do more of your own research as well!

Regardless of our own personal experiences, we both understand the difficulty in *mentally* overcoming long-held beliefs about what is *good* or *bad* for us. At this point, there are many people who now believe ~ as we ourselves did at various points ~ that *all* sugar is bad, including fruit. In fact, many consider fructose to be especially 'toxic' however as Ray Peat explains, fructose is required in at least equal amounts to glucose to optimize the use of sugar for fueling our brain, and in deed, our lives. Most fruits and honey are an ideal balance of both fructose and glucose, maple syrup is mostly sucrose, which is a 50/50 blend of fructose and glucose, while grains and starchy foods contain only glucose.

We Need More Than High Vitality Foods To Thrive

Many spiritual teachings emphasize the need to have a *burning desire* in life. You can always identify those who are passionately engaged in meaningful pursuits. They seem to be tapped into an endless reservoir of energy, rarely complaining about any aches and pains. Having gratitude, and loving your life may be the most potent panacea for experiencing optimal health. Let your food nurture your nature so you can focus on sharing your gifts in meaningful and rewarding ways.

Long-lived populations have been studied to determine what elements help promote their longer than average life spans. It is clear that a few key reasons likely include eating fresh locally produced foods, living among a close-knit community of extended family members, and those of shared values, remaining physically active, expressing gratitude, while also maintaining greater life balance.

Studies indicate that social isolation, especially as we age, can lead to increased physical and mental decline, remedied when both the young and old come together to work on projects, and share companionship. And while many rural Americans struggle financially, especially compared to their urban and suburban counterparts, having strong social networks improves quality of life. "Almost three-quarters (73%) of rural Americans rate the overall quality of life in their local community as excellent or good. And a majority (62%) are optimistic that people like them can make an impact on their local community."[1] In small towns, neighbors help each other. That provides a level of 'social security' many of us in larger urban areas may be missing, despite higher average incomes.

Sociologist Robert Putnam, author of **BOWLING ALONE** interviewed 30,000 people in neighborhoods across the United States to determine 'social capital' and discussed his findings in a paper entitled, E PLURIBUS UNUM: DIVERSITY AND COMMUNITY IN THE 21ST CENTURY. Putnam was surprised to discover that "In the most diverse communities, neighbors trust one another about half as much as they do in the most homogenous settings." Instead, they tended to withdraw more into their shell, 'like a turtle' and spend more time "unhappily in front of the television" while participating less in community

---

[1] NPR Poll: Many Rural Americans Struggle With Financial Insecurity, Access To Health Care, May 21, 2019 https://www.npr.org/sections/health-shots/2019/05/21/725059882/poll-many-rural-americans-struggle-with-financial-insecurity-access-to-health-ca

affairs, with less charitable contributions, volunteering, voting, and more.[2,3,4,5]

As humans, we require adequate fresh air, sunshine, and shared kinship and fellowship in order to truly thrive. Instead, many now work hard yet barely make ends meet. Parents are busier than ever, working and shuttling children to a myriad of after school activities. (Nothing like I recall in my younger days. I walked to and from school, and played outdoors!) Our current culture is encouraged to maintain a hyper-focus on material pursuits, and superficial, fleeting pleasures. Distractions abound putting people in sensory overload. In addition to a plethora of unhealthful foods many now consume ~ including lab-made *foods* (I use that term lightly) touted as 'healthy'~ we are inundated with other forms of 'food' ~ that are toxic to our mental, emotional, and spiritual development. Our true biological, human needs are being edged out, including spiritual pursuits that would otherwise provide far greater life balance.

---

[2] Stanford Social Innovation Review, Notes on Robert Putnam's "E Pluribus Unum: Diversity and Community in the Twenty-First Century"By Albert Ruesga, August 20. 2007, https://ssir.org/articles/entry/notes_on_robert_putnams_diversity_and_community_in_the_twenty_first_century

[3] Wiley Online Library, E Pluribus Unum: Diversity and Community in the Twenty-First Century The 2006 Johan Skytte Prize Lecture, 15 June, 2007, https://onlinelibrary.wiley.com/doi/abs/10.1111/j.1467-9477.2007.00176.x

[4] http://www.edwest.co.uk/uncategorized/does-diversity-makes-us-unhappy/

[5] Does Diversity Create Distrust? Scientific American, https://www.scientificamerican.com/article/does-diversity-create-distrust/

All this has caused many of us to act and live in ways that run counter to our true nature. The result is what we are now witnessing: More and more people, especially women, are taking antidepressants, and more and more people are riddled with anxiety, overdosing on drugs, committing suicide, not sleeping well, and feeling isolated and alone. That is in addition to increasing rates of obesity, diabetes and cardiovascular disease, and many other diseases of 'civilization' with a decreased ability to do basic physical activities. In short, it would appear that far *too few* people, relatively speaking, are living a high vitality life! Our modern 'health care' system does not address the root of what ails us. Bottom line, living *counter* to our true nature leads to suffering and dis-ease, whether we are consciously aware of this or not.

We believe there is a better way. Many things may seem 'broken' to the seasoned observer ~ including current agendas bent on vilifying, taxing, and replacing real foods, especially beef, dairy and eggs, with fake, lab-made alternatives. Claims are made that meat is bad for you, and bad for the environment, but these claims ~ while they may sound convincing, and even dire ~ are not backed by solid science.

It has become very clear to us that while we were briefly caught up in the vegan ideology and propaganda, animal foods are essential for achieving optimal health. There are many important nutrients only found in an absorbable form in animal foods. While Don's first edition of **THE HYPERCARNIVORE DIET** was highly referenced, he is making some essential updates after an even more thorough look at research missed the first time around.

We hope you will benefit from the fruits or our labor, and indulge in the meats and sweets that most appeal to you. Enjoy summer's bounty of fresh fruit, a bowl of ice cream, or warm milk and honey before bed. And do eat meat! It really is good for you, as you will learn in the next chapter!

From the depths of our hearts, Don and I wish you all a healthy, sweet, high vitality life!

2 - WHY A HIGH VITALITY DIET?

"A major part of the diet should be milk, cheese, eggs, shellfish, fruits, and coconut oil." ~Ray Peat

MEATS & SWEETS ~ A HIGH VITALITY DIET is a way of eating in harmony with your Nature. It emphasizes eating nutrient-dense foods to support an efficient and regenerative metabolism.

What Foods Best Support Human Nature?

Nature has endowed every species with equipment capable of acquiring the types of foods that the individuals of that species require to achieve their genetic potentials. We call this equipment the Food Acquisition Equipment (FAE).

Humans have FAE designed to lead us to the consumption of a diet rich in fruits (Nature's sweets) and meats. The human FAE includes:

Vision: The visual cortex dominates the human brain, whereas the olfactory cortex dominates the brain of classic carnivores like dogs and cats. Emphasis on vision supports gathering plants, which have little odor but distinct shapes and colors (particularly in flowers and fruits), whereas emphasis on smell supports hunting animals, which have distinct odors but camouflage coloration.

According to Stanley Coren, a professor of psychology and expert on human-dog interactions, humans have a visual system very specifically adapted to a diet based on gathering various types of fruits; whereas the dog has a sensory system naturally, primarily, and very specifically adapted to hunting animals:

"Because humans evolved from tree-dwelling primates, we needed eyes that could see colors (to pick out ripe fruit and nuts from among the leaves of trees), good visual acuity (to see small nuts and berries), and good depth perception (so that we would not misjudge the distance between branches and fall to the ground). The ancestors of dogs were primarily hunters and meat eaters that were adapted to run swiftly on the ground to pursue prey that might be distant but still within chasing range. Canines are also 'crepuscular,' meaning they are usually active at dusk and dawn and are more comfortable than humans when operating in dim light. The type of eye needed for twilight and nighttime activity requires sensitivity to low levels of brightness, but perception of color is really not very important."[6]

Animals primarily adapted to hunting need a good ability to discriminate moving objects (prey). Cats and dogs have relatively poor visual acuity compared to humans, but a greater ability to discriminate moving objects.[7]

---

[6] Coren S. How Dogs Think: Understanding the Canine Mind. New York, Free Press, 2004. 17.

[7] Ibid, pages 26 and 29.

Sweet taste: All great apes, including humans, have taste receptors uniquely adapted to detecting fructose and sucrose, carbohydrates found concentrated in fruits. These sweet receptors emerged in the hominoid primate lineage more than thirty-five million years ago, and probably played a critical role in support of primate brain evolution by improving food search efficiency and dietary selection of sugar- and energy-rich fruits.[8]

---

[8] Nofre C, Tinti JM, and D. Glaser D. Evolution of the Sweetness Receptor in Primates. II. Gustatory Responses of Non-human Primates to Nine Compounds Known to be Sweet in Man. Chem. Senses 21: 747-762, 1996.

Compared to humans, cats and dog have far fewer total taste receptors,[9] a general loss of taste receptor function,[10] and lack sweet taste receptors.[11, 12, 13] These carnivores have taste receptors primarily tuned to amino acids from meat, whereas many studies show that humans describe raw meat as essentially bland, having no flavor to speak of (if you've eaten raw meat you know this is true).[14, 15]

---

[9] Coren S. How Dogs Think: Understanding the Canine Mind. New York, Free Press, 2004. 82.

[10] Jiang P, Josue J, Li X, et al. Major taste loss in carnivorous animals. PNAS USA 2012 Mar 27;109(13):4956-61.

[11] Monell Chemical Senses Center (2012, March 12). Extensive taste loss found in mammals: Feeding preferences shaped by taste receptors. ScienceDaily. Retrieved September 16, 2013, from http://www.sciencedaily.com/releases/2012/03/120312152639.htm

[12] Li X, Li W, Wang H, et al. Cats lack a sweet taste receptor. J Nutr. 2006 July; 136(7 Suppl): 1932S–1934S.

[13] Callaway E. Carnivores have evolved to pick meat over sweets. Scientific American, March 12, 2012.

[14] Speth JD. The Paleoanthropology and Archaeology of Big-Game Hunting. Interdisciplinary Contributions to Archaeology, DOI 10.1007/978-1-4419-6733-6_8, Springer Science+Business Media, LLC 2010. 119-120.

[15] Mottram DS, Koutsidis G, Oruna-Concha M, et al. Analysis of Important Flavor Precursors in Meat. In: Deibler KD, Delwiche J, Handbook of Flavor Characterization: Sensory Analysis, Chemistry, and Physiology. Marcel Dekker, New York, NY, 463-472.

Carnivores (e.g. dogs, cats) have specific taste for water[16] but not for salt[17,18], while humans have a taste for salt but not for water. A carnivore needs a specific taste for water but not for salt because meat is high in sodium but low in water; whereas a frugivore needs a specific taste for salt but not for water because fruits are high in water but low in sodium.

Saliva: Fruits contain large amounts of phenols/flavonoids known as tannins. Some people call tannins antinutrients, because they bind and reduce the digestibility and bioavailability of dietary proteins.

Animals adapted to tannin-rich foods produce salivary proline-rich proteins (PRPs) which help an animal extract nutritional value from plant foods by binding with dietary tannins. Studies of mice and rats have shown that PRPs neutralize the detrimental effects of tannins.[19]

---

[16] Coren, op. cit., 86.

[17] Coren, op. cit., 83.

[18] Yu S and Morris JG. Sodium Requirement of Adult Cats for Maintenance Based on Plasma Aldosterone. J Nutr 1999 Feb 1;129(2):419-423.

[19] Mehanso H, Butler LG, Carlson DM. Dietary Tannins and Salivary Proline-Rich Proteins: Interactions, Induction, and Defense Mechanisms. Annual Review of Nutrition 1987 Jul 1;7(1):423-40.

Humans have a salivary PRP content consistent with an evolved physiological commitment to to a tannin/phenol-rich diet. About 70% of the proteins in human saliva consist of PRPs.[20] Some authors go so far as to suggest that humans have a "taste" for tannins since we seem to even seek out and prefer foods with a certain level of tannins, such as tea, red wine, beer, chocolate, smoked foods, herbs, and spices.[21]

Evidently, we are well adapted to tannins. Also, we have evidence that tannins (polyphenols, flavonoids) act as important chemopreventers of infectious and chronic diseases in humans; they have antioxidant, anti-inflammatory, vasoprotective, vasodilatory, antibacterial, antiallergic, hepatoprotective, antithrombotic, antiviral, neuroprotective, and anticarcinogenic effects.[22, 23]

Digestive Tract: Frugivore and carnivore guts are in many ways similar because both rely on enzymatic digestion of food, not fermentation as found in herbivores. Our gut has proportions and absorptive surface area indicative of a flexible frugivorous carnivore, or carnivorous frugivore.

---

[20] Mehanso H, et al, op. cit., 424.

[21] Ibid., 424.

[22] Habauzit V, Morand C. Evidence for a protective effect of polyphenols-containing foods on cardiovascular health: an update for clinicians. Ther Adv Chronic Dis 2012 Mar;3(2):87-106. PMC3513903.

[23] Soobrattee MA, Bahorun T, Aruoma OI. Chemopreventive actions of polyphenolic compounds in cancer. Biofactors 2006 Jan 1:27(1):19-35. 21.

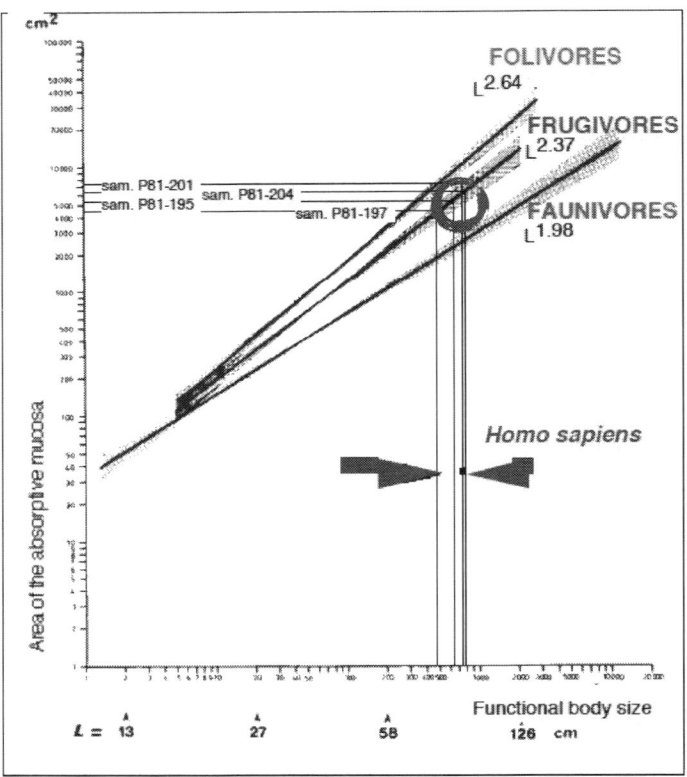

Figure 1: Ratio of absorptive mucosa to body size in 180 mammals including 117 primates. Source: Hladik CM, Pasquet P. The human adaptations to meat eating: a reappraisal. Human Evolution, Springer Verlag, 2002;17: 199-206.

Faunivores (carnivores) have less gut absorptive area per unit body size, herbivores more, and frugivores lie in between (Figure 1). Herbivores need the most gut absorption area because non-fruit plants have very low energy density. Carnivores need the least absorptive area because meat and fat have highest energy density. Frugivores need an intermediate absorptive area because fruits have an intermediate energy density. Humans have a ratio of absorptive mucosa to body size that most closely matches the frugivore ratio (Figure 1). This frugivorous gut that gives us our extreme dietary flexibility so we can eat both easily digested plants and meat.[24]

Our ratio of cranial capacity:body mass is also most similar to the highly frugivorous monkeys and apes, whose brain:body ratio far exceeds any non-primate terrestrial carnivore (Figure 2).

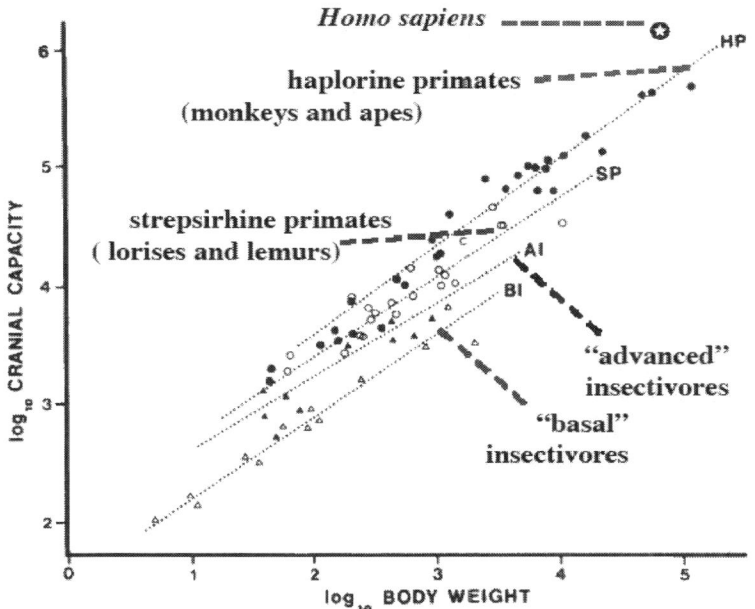

Figure 2: Ratio of cranial capacity to body weight in primates; insectivores are carnivores. Source: Hladik CM, Pasquet P. The human adaptations to meat eating: a reappraisal. Human Evolution, Springer Verlag, 2002;17: 199-206.

---

[24] Hladik CM, Pasquet P. The human adaptations to meat eating: a reappraisal. Human Evolution, Springer Verlag, 2002;17: 199-206.

Our gut proportions are most like that of the large brained spider monkey which gets on average 75% of its sustenance from fruits[25] (Table 1.1).

Table 1.1: Stomach, small intestine, cecum and colon proportions in five primate species

Species	Stomach	Small Intestine	Cecum	Colon
Spider monkey[1]	13	62	8	18
Orangutan	17	28	3	54
Gorilla[2]	25	14	7	53
Chimpanzee[2]	20	23	5	52
Human[2]	17	62	Vestigial Appendix	20

1. Milton K. Food choice and digestive strategies of two sympatric primate species. The American Naturalist, April 1981; 117 (4): 496-505.
2. Milton K. Primate diets and gut morphology: Implications for Hominid Evolution. In Harris M (ed.), Food And Evolution: Toward a Theory of Human Food Habits, Temple University Press, 1989. 93-116.

---

[25] Milton K. Food choice and digestive strategies of two sympatric primate species. The American Naturalist, April 1981; 117 (4): 496-505. <nature.berkeley.edu/miltonlab/pdfs/foodchoice.pdf>

Like the spider monkey, the majority of our gut volume is concentrated in the small intestine. Gorillas, chimpanzees, and orangutans subsist on lower ratios of fruit and higher intakes of leaves. To process this high fiber diet they have the majority of their gut volumes in the colon and cecum where they ferment the leaves to extract energy from the plant fiber.

We are about the same size as chimps, but with a larger brain, and smaller gut, with a small volume colon and virtually no cecum, which rules out fermentation of fiber from leaves as a major energy source for us. We need a diet with a little higher energy density and we get it via consumption of more meat than any other primate.

Consequently, we have some gut features indicating a specialization in consuming a fair amount of meat. The most important of these are our highly acidic stomach and our highly developed gall bladder.

Table 1.2: Stomach pH of various species

Common name	Diet/digestion type	Stomach pH
Colobus monkey	plantivore/foregut	6.3
Sheep	plantivore/hindgut	4.7
Dog	scavenger	4.5
Ox	herbivore/foregut	4.2
Horse	herbivore/hindgut	4.4
Cat	carnivore	3.6
Baboon	omnivore	3.7
Crab-eating macaque	omnivore	3.6
Skyes monkey	omnivore	3.4
Snowy owl	carnivore	2.5
Bottlenose dolpin	carnivore	2.3
Cynomolgus monkey	omnivore	2.1
Rabbit	plantivore/hindgut; eats feces	1.9
Grey falcon	scavenger	1.8
American bittern	scavenger	1.7
Red tailed hawk	scavenger	1.8
Swanson's hawk	scavenger	1.8
Human	**carnivore**	**1.5**
Ferret	carnivore	1.5
Wandering albatross	scavenger	1.5
Possum	scavenger	1.5

Source: Beasley DE, Koltz AM, Lambert JE, et al., "The Evolution of Stomach Acidity and Its Relevance to the Human Microbiome," PLOS One 2015 July 29.

Our stomach produces an extremely low pH of 1.5, making it more acidic than any other primate, considerably more acidic than most carnivores and "omnivores," and most similar to carrion feeders,[26] indicating a strong adaptation to eating meat (see Table 1.2).

Since carnivores eat intermittent meals rich in fat, with very few exceptions Nature has provided them with very well-developed gall bladders. This enables them to efficiently digest their naturally high-fat diet, and to have regular bowel movements.

---

[26] Beasley DE, Koltz AM, Lambert JE, et al., "The Evolution of Stomach Acidity and Its Relevance to the Human Microbiome," PLOS One 2015 July 29. <http://journals.plos.org/plosone/article?id=10.1371/journal.pone.0134116>

An exclusively fruit-based diet would be very low in fat in comparison to a diet including some meat. In humans who eat a very low fat diet, the gall bladder does not completely empty, giving rise to gall stone formation and constipation.[27, 28] In humans, very low fat, high carbohydrate plant-based diets may increase the risk for gall bladder stones.[29]

This evidence indicates that Nature designed our gall bladder for a diet containing more fat than found in other primate diets. In Nature, only regular meat consumption can provide enough fat to require the type of gall bladder development we have. It should be noted that the natural diet of chimpanzees is estimated at 2.5% of dry weight.[30] Consequently even a diet that is only 15-25% fat by dry weight (typical in Western nations) is very high in fat in comparison to other primates' diets.

---

[27] Festi D, Colecchia A, Larocca A, Villanova N, Mazzella G, Petroni ML, RomanoF, Roda E. Review: low caloric intake and gall-bladder motor function. Aliment Pharmacol Ther. 2000 May;14 Suppl 2:51-3. Review. PubMed PMID: 10903004.

[28] Stokes CS, Gluud LL, Casper M, Lammert F. Ursodeoxycholic Acid and Diets Higher in Fat Prevent Gallbladder Stones During Weight Loss: A Meta-analysis of Randomized Controlled Trials. Clin Gastroenter and Hepat 2014;12:1090-1100. <http://www.cghjournal.org/article/S1542-3565(13)01837-5/pdf>

[29] Tsai C-J, Leitzmann MF, Willett WC, Giovannucci EL. Dietary carbohydrates and glycaemic load and the incidence of symptomatic gall stone disease in men. *Gut*. 2005;54(6):823-828. doi:10.1136/gut.2003.031435. <https://www.ncbi.nlm.nih.gov/pmc/articles/PMC1774557/>

[30] Finch CE and Stanford CB. Meat-Adaptive Genes and the Evolution of Slower Aging in Humans. The Quarterly Review of Biology 2004 Mar;79(1): 3-50. 19.

So, to reiterate, we have the guts of a frugivore that is also highly adapted to eating meat and fat. Nature designed us for eating a diet composed of some combination of meats and low fiber, high sugar plants ~ fruits, or, as we say, meats and sweets.

It is our dietary flexibility that creates so much confusion in diet and nutrition research and the conflict between the advocates of plant-based and animal-based diets. Since we have a highly flexible gut that can adapt to diets with widely varying proportions of plant and animal matter, experiments can easily be designed to prove that we do well on either highly plant based or highly animal based diets. It is up to each individual to discover their personal sweet spot, or ideal ratio of fruits and meats.

Why We Need Meats

Unlike animal proteins, plant proteins do not have the balance of amino acids that we require (this is why plant proteins are said to be incomplete, whereas animal proteins are said to be complete). Plant proteins do not contain the amino acid taurine, for which we probably have a dietary requirement.[31, 32, 33, 34, 35]

We may also require animal protein to obtain adequate amounts of the amino acids methionine and choline. A 2000 study found low methionine levels typical in vegans and vegetarians.[36] Low methionine intake has several harmful or accelerated aging effects, including:

---

31 Laidlaw SA et al., "Plasma and urine taurine levels in vegans," Am J Clin Nutr 1988 Apr;47(4):660-3.

32 Eishorbagy A et al., "Amino acid changes during transition to a vegan diet supplemented with fish in healthy humans," Eur J Nut 2016 Jun. <http://link.springer.com/article/10.1007%2Fs00394-016-1237-6>

33 Rana SK, Sanders TA, "Taurine concentrations in the diet, plasma, urine and breast milk of vegans compared with omnivores," Br J Nutr 1986 Jul;56(1):17-27.

34 Naismith DJ, Rana SK, Emery PW, "Metabolism of taurine during reproduction in women," Hum Nutr Clin Nutr 1987 Jan;41(1):37-45.

35 McCarty MF, "Sub-optimal taurine status may promote platelet hyperaggregability in vegetarians," Med Hypotheses 2004;63(3):426-33.

36 Krajcovicová-Kudláčková M, Blazícek P, Kopcová J, Béderová A, Babinská K, "Homocysteine levels in vegetarians versus omnivores," Ann Nutr Metab 2000;44(3):135-8. PubMed PMID: 11053901.

- reduced levels of sulfur, which impairs detoxification and connective tissue repair[37]
- reduced levels of glutathione, compromising antioxidant defenses and promoting inflammation[38]
- inflammation and deterioration of gut structure[39]
- impaired immune function and recovery from injury[40]
- greying of hair; methionine depletion leads to a buildup of hydrogen peroxide in hair follicles which causes loss of hair color[41, 42]
- increased risk for venous thrombosis[43]

---

[37] Nimni ME, Han B, Cordoba F. Are we getting enough sulfur in our diet? *Nutrition & Metabolism*. 2007;4:24. doi:10.1186/1743-7075-4-24. <https://www.ncbi.nlm.nih.gov/pmc/articles/PMC2198910/>

[38] Ibid.

[39] Ruth MR, Field CJ. The immune modifying effects of amino acids on gut-associated lymphoid tissue. J Animal Sci and Biotech 2013;4:27. <https://jasbsci.biomedcentral.com/articles/10.1186/2049-1891-4-27>

[40] Grimble RF. The Effects of Sulfur Amino Acid Intake on Immune Function in Humans. J Nutr 2006 June;136(6):1660S-1665S. <https://doi.org/10.1093/jn/136.6.1660S>

[41] Wood JM, Decker H, Hartmann H, et al. Senile hair graying: H2O2-mediated oxidative stress affects human hair color by blunting methionine sulfoxide repair. FASEB J. 2009 Jul;23(7):2065-75. doi: 10.1096/fj.08-125435. Epub 2009 Feb 23. PubMed PMID: 19237503.

[42] Schallreuter KU, Salem MM, Hasse S, Rokos H. The redox--biochemistry of human hair pigmentation. Pigment Cell Melanoma Res. 2011 Feb;24(1):51-62. doi: 10.1111/j.1755-148X.2010.00794.x. Epub 2010 Dec 1. PubMed PMID: 20958953.

[43] Keijzer MB, den Heijer M, Borm GF, et al. Low fasting methionine concentration as a novel risk factor for recurrent venous thrombosis. Thromb Haemost. 2006 Oct;96(4):492-7. PubMed PMID: 17003928.

- increased risk of infertility[44]

We also need to eat meat to get adequate dietary choline. Choline is essential for a number of functions including neurotransmitter synthesis, cell structure, and methylation. Requirements are increased during pregnancy and lactation to support neurological development in children. Choline deficiency plays a roll in liver disease, poor offspring, cognitive function and neurological disorders. A 2019 study provided evidence that a lifelong high intake of choline (4.5 times the recommended adequate intake) might prevent Alzheimer's disease.[45]

Plant foods are poor sources of choline. The best sources of choline are beef liver (431mg per 100g) and eggs with the yolks (226mg per 100g). Aside from human milk, the next best sources include beef steak (104mg/100g), salmon (90.4mg/100g), pork chops (78.2mg/100g) and chicken breast (61.8mg/100g). (All measurements listed are based on cooked foods.)

---

[44] Grandison RC, Piper MDW, Partridge L. Amino acid imbalance explains extension of lifespan by dietary restriction in *Drosophila*. *Nature* 2009;462(7276): 1061-1064. doi:10.1038/nature08619.

[45] Arizona State University. "Common nutrient supplementation may hold the answers to combating Alzheimer's disease." ScienceDaily. ScienceDaily, 27 September 2019. <www.sciencedaily.com/releases/2019/09/190927122526.htm>.

An adult needs the amount of choline found in 2 egg yolks daily to obtain the recommended adequate intake (425-550 mg/d). Egg white omelettes are touted as 'heart healthy' on many restaurant menus, but in truth, the real nutritional value to eggs is in the yolk.

Archaeological evidence of iron and vitamin B12 deficiency diseases in the bones of a 2 year-old child dated to 1.5 million years ago indicates that by that time humans in their natural habitat (our ancestors) already had a dietary requirement for meat from grass-eating animals to prevent childhood iron and vitamin B12 deficiency diseases.[46]

---

46 Domínguez-Rodrigo M, Pickering TR, Diez-Martín F, Mabulla A, Musiba C, Trancho G, et al. (2012) Earliest Porotic Hyperostosis on a 1.5-Million-Year-Old Hominin, Olduvai Gorge, Tanzania. PLoS ONE 7(10): e46414. doi:10.1371/journal.pone.0046414<https://www.ncbi.nlm.nih.gov/pmc/articles/PMC3463614/>

Impoverished children in developing countries who do not get adequate animal source foods (meat, eggs, milk) in their diets suffer from micronutrient malnutrition that causes growth stunting, lower intelligence, lethargy, poor attention, and greater rates and severity of infections.[47] Children raised in Europe on unsupplemented vegan diets have a high risk of deficiencies of vitamins B12 and D with consequences including stunted growth, rickets, and impaired cognitive capacity, with the latter persisting despite subsequent diet enrichment.[48, 49]

---

[47] Demmet MW, Young MM, Sensenig RL. Animal Source Foods to Improve Micronutrient Nutrition and Human Function in Developing Countries. Providing Micronutrients through Food-Based Solutions: A Key to Human and National Development. J Nutr 2003;133:3879S-3885S. Accessed online on Dec 12, 2017 from: <http://jn.nutrition.org/content/133/11/3879S.full.pdf>

[48] Di Genova T, Guyda H. Infants and children consuming atypical diets: Vegetarianism and macrobiotics. *Paediatrics & Child Health*. 2007;12(3):185-188. <https://www.ncbi.nlm.nih.gov/pmc/articles/PMC2528709/>

[49] Roberts IF, West RJ, Ogilvie D, Dillon MJ. Malnutrition in infants receiving cult diets: a form of child abuse. *British Medical Journal*. 1979;1(6159):296-298. <https://www.ncbi.nlm.nih.gov/pmc/articles/PMC1597704/?page=1>

People who avoid animal protein develop vitamin B12 deficiency even if they use typical vitamin B12 supplements; vitamin B12 deficiency and elevated plasma homocysteine have been found to be the "normal" state for vegans.[50] Vitamin supplements typically contain a poorly utilized form of B12 that is not found in plants, microbes or animal tissues, so they can't replace animal foods.[51]

Limiting meat intake also limits intake of highly bioavailable iron, zinc, selenium, and B-complex vitamins.[52, 53]

---

[50] Obersby D, Chappell DC, Dunnett A, Tsiami AA. Plasma total homocysteine status of vegetarians compared with omnivores: a systematic review and meta-analysis. Brit J Nutr 2013 Mar 14;109(5):785-94. <https://www.cambridge.org/core/journals/british-journal-of-nutrition/article/div-classtitleplasma-total-homocysteine-status-of-vegetarians-compared-with-omnivores-a-systematic-review-and-meta-analysisdiv/1754320C613E6CD7F9AED4EE60C421B5/core-reader>

[51] Kelly G. The Coenzyme Forms of Vitamin B12: Toward an Understanding of their Therapeutic Potential. Alternative Medicine Review 1997;2(6):459-471. Accessed Dec 12, 2017 from: <http://www.anaturalhealingcenter.com/documents/Thorne/articles/CoEnzymeB12.pdf>

[52] D.K. Layman, A. Arne Astrup, P.M. Clifton, H.J. Leidy, D. Paddon-Jones, S.M. Phillips, "The contrived association of dietary protein with mortality," Comments submitted to Cell Metabolism April 2, 2014 (2014) (Available at: http://www.cell.com/cell-metabolism/comments/S1550-4131(14)00062-X. Accessed March 29, 2017).

[53] Binnie MA, Barlow K, Johnson V, Harrison C, "Red meats: Time for a paradigm shift in dietary advice," Meat Science 2014 Nov;98(3):445-51. <http://www.sciencedirect.com/science/article/pii/S0309174014001922>

Advances in measuring protein needs suggest that the current RDA underestimates protein requirements by as much as 50%, and diets providing more protein than the RDA have been found beneficial for reducing excess energy (calorie) intake and cardiovascular risk factors.[54]

Benefits of Milk & Calcium

Milk is highly nutritious liquid meat. Milk is a rich source of very high quality animal protein and many essential nutrients, particularly calcium. Milk sugar (lactose) improves intestinal flora by increasing Bifidobacteria and reducing Bacterioides and Clostridia species.[55]

---

[54] Ibid.

[55] Singh RK, Chang HW, Yan D, et al. Influence of diet on the gut microbiome and implications for human health. *J Transl Med*. 2017;15(1):73. Published 2017 Apr 8. doi:10.1186/s12967-017-1175-y <https://www.ncbi.nlm.nih.gov/pmc/articles/PMC5385025/>

Calcium plays very important metabolic roles. Calcium activates proteins that produce cell movement, muscle contraction, nerve transmission, glandular secretion, blood clotting, and cell division and differentiation. Dietary or tissue calcium deficiency can cause or contribute to muscle cramping, edema, and skin disorders (psoriasis, atopic dermatitis).[56, 57, 58]

Calcium plays a critical role in the immune system and the killing of cancer cells is most likely calcium-dependent.[59] Calcium is required for maintaining intestinal integrity and prevention of leaky gut.[60]

---

[56] J M Belizán, J Villar; The relationship between calcium intake and edema-, proteinuria-, and hypertension-gestosis: an hypothesis, *The American Journal of Clinical Nutrition*, Volume 33, Issue 10, 1 October 1980, Pages 2202–2210, https://doi.org/10.1093/ajcn/33.10.2202

[57] Floriana Elsholz, Christian Harteneck, Walter Muller, Kristina Friedland. Calcium - a central regulator of keratinocyte differentiation in health and disease. European Journal of Dermatology. 2014;24(6):650-661. doi:10.1684/ejd.2014.2452

[58] Hung AKD. Severe hypocalcaemia as a cause of seemingly idiopathic bilateral lower limb oedema. *BMJ Case Reports*. 2014;2014:bcr2013201387. doi:10.1136/bcr-2013-201387. <https://www.ncbi.nlm.nih.gov/pmc/articles/PMC3902373/>

[59] Schwarz, E., Qu, B., & Hoth, M. (2013). Calcium, cancer and killing: The role of calcium in killing cancer cells by cytotoxic T lymphocytes and natural killer cells. Biochimica et Biophysica Acta (BBA) - Molecular Cell Research, 1833(7), 1603-1611.

[60] Gomes JMG, Costa JA, Alfenas RC. Could the beneficial effects of dietary calcium on obesity and diabetes control be mediated by changes in intestinal microbiota and integrity? *British Journal of Nutrition*. 2015;114(11):1756-1765. doi:10.1017/S0007114515003608

Wild primates and humans may give us some idea how much calcium we require. An early study of calcium metabolism in rhesus macaques concluded that a growing 3-kg monkey requires 150 mg calcium daily for each kg bodyweight.[61] Later studies found that this was not sufficient to prevent osteoporosis in the monkeys.[62] If human calcium requirements are similar, a 150 pound (68 kg) man would require 10 grams of calcium daily, an amount more than 10 times the current recommended daily allowance.

---

[61] National Academies: Nutrient Requirements of Nonhuman Primates: Second Revised Edition. National Academies Press, 2003. Chapter 6 Minerals. Page 95.

[62] Ibid.

Table 1.1: Estimated mineral intakes of wild howler monkeys compared to the human RDA.

Mineral	Total daily intake–7 kg adult monkey (mg)	RDA, 70 kg adult male (mg)
Calcium	4571	800
Phosphorus	728	800
Potassium	6419	2000
Sodium	182	500
Chloride	1778	750
Magnesium	1323	350
Iron	39	10
Manganese	18	5
Copper	3	3

Source: Milton K. Nutritional Characteristics of Wild Primate Foods, Nutrition 1995;15(6): 488-98. 493.

A 7 kg wild howler monkey consumes about 4600 mg of calcium daily (Table 1.1). Wild chimpanzees in their native habitat have diets that supply 80-100 mg calcium per 100 kcal, and both prehistoric and contemporary human hunter-gatherers have very high calcium intakes, in range of 70-80 mg per 100 kcal, or in excess of 2000 mg (50 mmol) per day.[63, 64] The latter obtained calcium from bones, egg shells, mineral-rich ground water and ashes. It is important to realize that hunter-gatherers had dietary customs that may at first glance seem inconsequential but on further examination played a very important role in meeting their nutritional needs. For example, the Navajo tribe habitually used an ash prepared from branches and needles of the juniper tree as a dietary seasoning and supplement. Just one teaspoon of this ash provides about as much calcium as a cup of cow milk (i.e. 300 mg).[65]

In contrast to wild primate and hunter-gatherer calcium intakes, the median intake for women in modern North America and European nations is less than 600 mg (15 mmol) per day.

---

[63] Heaney RP. The roles of calcium and vitamin D in skeletal health: an evolutionary perspective. <http://www.fao.org/docrep/W7336T/W7336T03.HTM>

[64] Eaton SB, Nelson DA: Calcium in evolutionary perspective. *Am. J. Clin. Nutr. 1991;* 54: 281S-287S.

[65] Whitney EN, Rolfes SR. Understanding Nutrition. 10th edition. Wadsworth/Thompson Learning 2005: 417.

A high protein diet increases calcium absorption but also increases urinary calcium excretion, and a person on a high protein diet probably needs a calcium intake of 20 mg per gram of dietary protein to protect the skeleton from depletion.[66, 67] Given that high protein and calcium intakes appear synergistic in promoting bone health and characteristic of preagricultural diets, it appears likely that we are by nature adapted to a diet that is high in both protein and calcium.[83, 84, 86]

Since a **HIGH VITALITY DIET** may provide 100-150 grams of protein daily, this would translate to a requirement for 2000-4000 mg calcium daily, which remarkably corresponds to the estimated calcium intakes of wild chimpanzees and hunter-gatherers.

---

[66] Gaffney-Stomberg E, Sun B, Cucchi CE, et al. The Effect of Dietary Protein on Intestinal Calcium Absorption in Rats. *Endocrinology*. 2010;151(3):1071-1078. doi:10.1210/en.2009-0744.

[67] Heaney RP: Excess Dietary Protein May Not Adversely Affect Bone, *The Journal of Nutrition*, Volume 128, Issue 6, 1 June 1998, Pages 1054–1057, https://doi.org/10.1093/jn/128.6.1054

Most people can tolerate fermented dairy products.[68, 69, 70] Milk products are excellent food sources of calcium. Whole milk and yogurt provide about 275 mg of calcium per 8 ounce serving, and aged cheeses provide about 200 mg calcium per 1 ounce serving. Two or more servings (serving = 8 oz milk or yogurt, 1 oz cheese) daily will satisfy requirements.

---

[68] Brown-Riggs C. Nutrition and Health Disparities: The Role of Dairy in Improving Minority Health Outcomes. Edberg M, Hayes BE, Rice VM, Tchounwou PB, eds. *International Journal of Environmental Research and Public Health*. 2016;13(1):28. doi:10.3390/ijerph13010028. <https://www.ncbi.nlm.nih.gov/pmc/articles/PMC4730419/>

[69] Jarvis JK, Miller GD. Overcoming the barrier of lactose intolerance to reduce health disparities. *Journal of the National Medical Association*. 2002;94(2):55-66. <https://www.ncbi.nlm.nih.gov/pmc/articles/PMC2594135/>

[70] Gaskin DJ, Ilich JZ. Lactose maldigestion revisited: Diagnosis, Prevalence in Ethnic Minorities, and Dietary Recommendations to Overcome it. Am J Lifestyle Med 2009 May 1;3(3):7.

Moderating Meat Intake

As discussed above, meat, eggs and milk supply critical nutrients not richly supplied by fruits. However, all nutrients have an optimal intake level. If you consume too little, you develop deficiencies; if you consume too much, you develop toxicity. Meat is a very concentrated source of critical nutrients that plants either lack or very poorly supply, including fat, phosphorus, and methionine. We need to eat some meat to avoid deficiencies of these nutrients. On the other hand, since meat is very highly nutrient dense, we can consume excesses of some nutrients – including fats, phosphorus, protein and methionine – if we consume too much meat.

Meat is a rich source of fat, and although consuming some saturated animal fat can be beneficial to health, an excess may be harmful. Bacteria in our guts produce endotoxin, which produces inflammation if absorbed into the blood. High fat meals increase endotoxin absorption by up to 50%.[71, 72, 73, 74, 75]

---

[71] Erridge C, Attina T, Spickett CM, Webb DJ. A high-fat meal induces low-grade endotoxemia: evidence of a novel mechanism of postprandial inflammation. Am JClin Nutr. 2007 Nov;86(5):1286-92. PubMed PMID: 17991637. <https://www.ncbi.nlm.nih.gov/pubmed/17991637>

[72] Vors C, Drai J, Pineau G, et al. Emulsifying dietary fat modulates postprandial endotoxemia associated with chylomicronemia in obese men: a pilot randomized crossover study. *Lipids Health Dis*. 2017;16(1):97. Published 2017 May 25. doi: 10.1186/s12944-017-0486-6

[73] López-Moreno J, García-Carpintero S, Jimenez-Lucena R, Haro C, Rangel-Zúñiga OA, Blanco-Rojo R, Yubero-Serrano EM, Tinahones FJ, Delgado-Lista J, Pérez-Martínez P, Roche HM, López-Miranda J, Camargo A. Effect of Dietary Lipids on Endotoxemia Influences Postprandial Inflammatory Response. J Agric Food Chem. 2017 Sep 6;65(35):7756-7763. doi: 10.1021/acs.jafc.7b01909. Epub 2017 Aug 22. PubMed PMID: 28793772.

[74] Ghanim H, Abuaysheh S, Sia CL, et al. Increase in plasma endotoxin concentrations and the expression of Toll-like receptors and suppressor of cytokine signaling-3 in mononuclear cells after a high-fat, high-carbohydrate meal: implications for insulin resistance. *Diabetes Care*. 2009;32(12):2281–2287. doi: 10.2337/dc09-0979 <https://www.ncbi.nlm.nih.gov/pmc/articles/PMC2782991/>

[75] Deopurkar R, Ghanim H, Friedman J, et al. Differential effects of cream, glucose, and orange juice on inflammation, endotoxin, and the expression of Toll-like receptor-4 and suppressor of cytokine signaling-3. *Diabetes Care*. 2010;33(5): 991–997. doi:10.2337/dc09-1630.

One study found that meals high in saturated fats were so effective at increasing endotoxin absorption that "a person eating three high-SFA meals each day may encounter endotoxin levels that remain perpetually high, since refeeding may increase the levels."[76]

A diet too rich in fat may also adversely impact the gut microbiome. Diets high in saturated fat increase the proportion of Faecalibacterium prausnitzii, and lard-enriched diets increase Bacterioides (the species that contributes most to endotoxin) and Bilophila.[77]

---

[76] Harte AL, Varma MC, Tripathi G, et al. High fat intake leads to acute postprandial exposure to circulating endotoxin in type 2 diabetic subjects. *Diabetes Care*. 2012;35(2):375–382. doi:10.2337/dc11-1593. <https://www.ncbi.nlm.nih.gov/pmc/articles/PMC3263907/>

[77] Singh RK, Chang HW, Yan D, et al. Influence of diet on the gut microbiome and implications for human health. *J Transl Med*. 2017;15(1):73. Published 2017 Apr 8. doi:10.1186/s12967-017-1175-y

Meat has a high amount of phosphorus and a high ratio of phosphorus to calcium. Although we need to get this mineral from our diet, phosphorus toxicity causes extensive tissue damage and accelerates aging.[78, 79] Excess phosphate produces fatigue, heart failure, movement dis-coordination, hypogonadism, infertility, vascular calcification, emphysema, cancer, osteoporosis, and atrophy of skin, muscle, intestine, thymus and spleen. An absolute phosphorus intake greater than 1400 mg per day and a dietary phosphorus density greater than 0.35 mg/kcal have both been associated with a doubled risk of all-cause mortality and a tripled risk of cardiovascular mortality.[80]

---

[78] Razzaque MS. Phosphate toxicity: new insights into an old problem. *Clin Sci (Lond)*. 2011;120(3):91–97. doi:10.1042/CS20100377.

[79] Ohnishi M, Razzaque MS. Dietary and genetic evidence for phosphate toxicity accelerating mammalian aging. FASEB J 2010; 24:3562-3571.

[80] Chang AR, Lazo M, Appel LJ, Gutiérrez OM, Grams ME. High dietary phosphorus intake is associated with all-cause mortality: results from NHANES III [published correction appears in Am J Clin Nutr. 2017 Apr;105(4):1021]. *Am J Clin Nutr*. 2014;99(2):320–327. doi:10.3945/ajcn.113.073148.

Excess intake of phosphorus exerts some of its negative effects by stimulating release of parathyroid hormone (PTH). Parathyroid hormone increases phosphate excretion, but it also has pro-inflammatory effects and is associated with increased mortality.[81, 82]

High phosphorus intake also suppresses activation of vitamin D.[83] This has a negative effect on calcium absorption and immune function.

A low dietary ratio of calcium to phosphorus raises parathyroid level, but increasing calcium intake to raise the ratio to at least 1:1 reduces the adverse effects of high phosphate.[84] Milk and milk products supply more calcium than phosphorus (ratio greater than 1:1).

---

[81] Cheng SP, Liu CL, Liu TP, Hsu YC, Lee JJ. Association between parathyroid hormone levels and inflammatory markers among US adults. *Mediators Inflamm.* 2014;2014:709024. doi:10.1155/2014/709024.

[82] Hui JY, Choi JW, Mount DB, Zhu Y, Zhang Y, Choi HK. The independent association between parathyroid hormone levels and hyperuricemia: a national population study. *Arthritis Res Ther.* 2012;14(2):R56. Published 2012 Mar 10. doi: 10.1186/ar3769.

[83] Portale AA, Halloran BP, Murphy MM, Morris RC Jr. Oral intake of phosphorus can determine the serum concentration of 1,25-dihydroxyvitamin D by determining its production rate in humans. *J Clin Invest.* 1986;77(1):7–12. doi: 10.1172/JCI112304.

[84] Kemi VE, Kärkkäinen MU, Karp HJ, Laitinen KA, Lamberg-Allardt CJ. Increased calcium intake does not completely counteract the effects of increased phosphorus intake on bone: an acute dose-response study in healthy females. Br J Nutr. 2008 Apr;99(4):832-9. Epub 2007 Oct 1. PubMed PMID: 17903344.

Fructose or sucrose (fruit, honey, maple syrup) increases excretion of phosphorus.[85] Therefore eating a lot of fruit and honey helps to protect against the potential adverse effects of eating meat.

As mentioned above, a dietary deficiency of the amino acid methionine, which is poorly supplied by plants, causes degenerative diseases. Nevertheless, too much methionine, from overconsumption of muscle meats, also may be harmful, unless counterbalanced by glycine intake.

---

[85] Milne DB, Nielsen FH. The interaction between dietary fructose and magnesium adversely affects macromineral homeostasis in men. J Am Coll Nutr. 2000 Feb; 19(1):31-7. PubMed PMID: 10682873.

Dietary studies have linked the absolute amount of dietary methionine (Met) and Met-derived homocysteine (Hcy) to reduced lifespan and age-related diseases.[86] Dietary Met restriction without kcalorie restriction extends lifespan in *Drosophila* and rodents[87], and selectively blocks cancer proliferation in humans because malignant cells have a greater Met dependency and requirement than normal cells.[88] Met-derived Hcy promotes atherosclerosis,[89] serves as a risk factor for cancer and a potential tumor marker[90], and may contribute to diabetic neuropathy[91], hypertension[92], and osteoporosis[93]. Evidence from epidemiological, experimental, and clinical trials suggests that Met-rich diets may promote atherosclerosis, cancer, diabetes,

---

[86] Schloss JV. On the Origin of Western Diet Pathologies. Nature Precedings 07/2010; DOI:http://hdl.handle.net/10101/npre.2010.4641.1.

[87] Grandison RC, Piper MDW, Partridge L. Amino acid imbalance explains extension of lifespan by dietary restriction in Drosophila. Nature 2009 Dec 24; 462:7276.

[88] Cellarier E, Durando X, Vasson MP, et al. Methionine dependency and cancer treatment. Cancer Treatment Reviews 2003;29:489-499.

[89] McCully KS. Homocysteine, vitamins, and vascular disease prevention. Am J Clin Nutr 2007 Nov;86(5):1563S-1568S.

[90] Wu LL, Wu JT. Hyperhomocysteinemia is a risk factor for cancer and a new potential tumor marker. Clinica Chimica Acta 2002 Aug 1;322(1):21-28.

[91] Wile DJ, Toth C. Association of Metformin, Elevated Homocysteine, and Methylmalonic Acid Levels and Clinically Worsened Diabetic Peripheral Neuropathy. Diabetes Care 2010 Jan 1;33(1):156-161.

[92] Stehouwer CDA, van Guldener C. Does Homocysteine Cause Hypertension? Clin Chem Lab Med 2003;41(11):1408-1411.

[93] Herrmann M, Widmann T, Herrmann W. Homocysteine - a newly recognized risk factor for osteoporosis. Clin Chem Lab Med 2005; 43(10):1111-1117.

hypertension, osteoporosis, and neurological diseases.[94, 95]

This information suggests that we may need to control or counter-balance tissue concentrations of methionine to achieve health and a long life span.

We can optimize intake of fat, phosphorus, protein and methionine by moderating meat intake. We can counter the ill effects of phosphorus by consuming adequate calcium (milk, calcium carbonate) and fruit, and we can counter the ill effects of methionine by consuming gelatin.

Gelatin

Our ancestors ate all parts of animals, not only the muscle meat. The vast majority of non-muscle protein in an animal carcass is collagen, which forms ~30% of all the protein in the body. Consequently, when our ancestors ate all edible parts of a carcass, they ate a large amount of collagen, from which we make gelatin.

---

[94] Campbell TC. Dietary protein, growth factors, and cancer. Am J Clin Nutr 2007 June; 85(6):1667.

[95] Campbell TC, Campbell TM II. The China Study: starling implications for diet, weight loss, and long term health. Dallas, TX: BenBella Books, Inc, 2005.

Gelatin is a rich source of glycine. Although not yet acknowledged by official bodies, a detailed account of all possible sources of glycine has demonstrated that typical diets and endogenous synthesis together provide only about 6 g/d, while requirements for all metabolic uses are *at least* 10 g/d greater than these supplies. Therefore glycine is a "conditionally essential" amino acid and we should eat foods rich in collagen or gelatin, or take a glycine supplement, in order to guarantee a healthy metabolism.[96]

Some people believe that a vegetarian diet supplies enough glycine without supplementation. However, when compared to meat-eaters, vegetarians excrete about twice as much 5-L-oxoproline, a marker for glycine deficiency, suggesting that a meat-free diet increases the risk of glycine deficiency.[97]

---

[96] Meléndez-Hevia E, De Paz-Lugo P, Cornish-Bowden A, Cárdenas ML. A weak link in metabolism: the metabolic capacity for glycine biosynthesis does not satisfy the need for collagen synthesis. J Biosci. 2009 Dec;34(6):853-72. PubMed PMID: 20093739. <https://www.ncbi.nlm.nih.gov/pubmed/20093739>

[97] Jackson AA, Persaud C, Meakins TS, Bundy R. Urinary Excretio of 5-L-Oxoproline (Pyroglutamic Acid) Is Increased in Normal Adults Consuming Vegetarian or Low Protein Diets. J Nutr 1996;126:2813-2822.

Glycine plays important roles in our metabolism. It forms 11.5% of total amino acids and 20% of amino acid nitrogen in body proteins. Protein synthesis, especially for collagen, uses 80% of whole-body glycine needs. It is needed for synthesis of glutathione, creatine, purines (DNA and RNA), heme, and serine. Through glycine-gated chloride channels, glycine modulates intracellular calcium levels, which regulates production of cytokines, generation of superoxide, and immune function. Glycine is an inhibitory neurotransmitter which improves sleep.

Glycine also increases insulin sensitivity.[98]

Glycine is required for synthesis of bile acids which are necessary for preventing gut bacterial overgrowth, maintaining bowel function, and digestion and absorption of dietary fat, particularly long-chain fatty acids, and fat soluble vitamins. It also mitigates the adverse effects of lipopolysaccharide (endotoxin), peptidoglycan polysaccharide, and peroxisome proliferators.[99]

---

[98] El-Hafidi M, Franco M, Ramírez AR, et al. Glycine Increases Insulin Sensitivity and Glutathione Biosynthesis and Protects against Oxidative Stress in a Model of Sucrose-Induced Insulin Resistance. *Oxid Med Cell Longev*. 2018;2018:2101562. Published 2018 Feb 21. doi:10.1155/2018/2101562. <https://www.ncbi.nlm.nih.gov/pmc/articles/PMC5841105/>

[99] Wang, W., Wu, Z., Dai, Z., Yang, Y., Wang, J., & Wu, G. (2013). Glycine metabolism in animals and humans: implications for nutrition and health. Amino Acids, 45(3), 463-477.

Glycine has anti-inflammatory, immunomodulatory and direct cytoprotective actions beneficial for inflammatory disorders. It acts on inflammatory cells to suppress formation of free radicals and inflammatory cytokines.[100]

Glycine also plays a special role in methionine metabolism, since it forms glycine-N-methyl transferase, the key enzyme in the only pathway for methionine clearance in mammals. Consequently, dietary glycine can block methionine toxicity. It is estimated that the optimal ratio of glycine to methionine for total diet is 3-4:1. To get this ratio on an animal-based diet one needs to consume 1 g of collagen for every 10 grams of non-collagen animal protein up to the 0.8 g/kg RDA and 1.5 g for every 10 g of non-collagen animal protein consumed beyond the RDA.

An 8% glycine diet has been shown to extend lifespan of animals with no evidence of impaired health.[101]

---

[100] Zhong Z, Wheeler MD, Li X, Froh M, Schemmer P, Yin M, Bunzendaul H, Bradford B, Lemasters JJ. L-Glycine: a novel antiinflammatory, immunomodulatory, and cytoprotective agent. Curr Opin Clin Nutr Metab Care. 2003 Mar;6(2):229-40. Review. PubMed PMID: 12589194.

[101] Miller RA, Harrison DE, Astle CM, et al. Glycine supplementation extends lifespan of male and female mice. *Aging Ceil*. 2019;18(3):e12953. doi:10.1111/acel.12953

For all these reasons we recommend liberal consumption of glycine-rich gelatin and collagen-rich animal products such as chicken feet, pig's ears, trotters, ox tail and so on.

The Sweets ~ Fruits and Honey

Fruit is rich in fructose, glucose, sucrose and minerals that support metabolism and health. A high intake of fruit protects against or improves intestinal flora[102] and many degenerative conditions[103] including:

- intestinal dysbiosis and colonic gastrointestinal diseases (e.g., constipation, irritable bowel syndrome, inflammatory bowel diseases, and diverticular disease)
- overweight and obesity
- cardiovascular diseases
- type 2 diabetes and metabolic syndrome
- colorectal and lung cancers
- premature and degenerative aging
- asthma and chronic obstructive pulmonary disease
- depression and other mental and behavioral disorders including autism spectrum disorder
- low bone mineral density (osteoporosis)

---

[102] Singh RK, Chang HW, Yan D, et al. Influence of diet on the gut microbiome and implications for human health. *J Transl Med*. 2017;15(1):73. Published 2017 Apr 8. doi:10.1186/s12967-017-1175-y <https://www.ncbi.nlm.nih.gov/pmc/articles/PMC5385025/>

[103] Dreher ML. Whole Fruits and Fruit Fiber Emerging Health Effects. *Nutrients*. 2018;10(12):1833. Published 2018 Nov 28. doi:10.3390/nu10121833

- seborrheic dermatitis

Honey intake reduces blood sugar levels and prevents excessive weight gain. It also improves lipid metabolism by reducing total cholesterol (TC), triglyceride (TG), low-density lipoprotein (LDL) and increasing high-density lipoprotein (HDL), which leads to decreased risk of atherogenesis. In addition, honey enhances insulin sensitivity that further stabilizes blood glucose levels and protects the pancreas from overstimulation brought on by insulin resistance. Furthermore, antioxidative properties of honey help in reducing oxidative stress. Lastly, honey protects the vasculature from endothelial dysfunction and remodeling.[104]

---

[104] Ramli NZ, Chin KY, Zarkasi KA, Ahmad F. A Review on the Protective Effects of Honey against Metabolic Syndrome. *Nutrients*. 2018;10(8):1009. Published 2018 Aug 2. doi:10.3390/nu10081009. <https://www.ncbi.nlm.nih.gov/pmc/articles/PMC6115915/>

Fruits and honey supply an abundance of fructose. Although current nutrition faddism would have people believe that any intake of fructose is harmful, in fact fructose is required for normal glucose metabolism and utilization.[105] Fructose and sucrose *increase* metabolic rate and thermogenesis and correct defects in carbohydrate oxidation and thermogenesis found in aging, obesity, and diabetes.[106,107, 108, 109] Fructose and sucrose produce a higher thermogenic effect (metabolic rate) than starch.[110] Fructose and sucrose prevent depression of metabolism when reducing food intake to lose body fat.[111]

---

[105] Laughlin MR. Normal roles for dietary fructose in carbohydrate metabolism. *Nutrients*. 2014;6(8):3117–3129. Published 2014 Aug 5. doi:10.3390/nu6083117

[106] Schwarz JM, Schutz Y, Froidevaux F, Acheson KJ, Jeanprêtre N, Schneider H, Felber JP, Jéquier E. Thermogenesis in men and women induced by fructose vs glucose added to a meal. Am J Clin Nutr. 1989 Apr;49(4):667-74. PubMed PMID: 2648796.

[107] Tappy L, Randin JP, Felber JP, Chiolero R, Simonson DC, Jequier E, DeFronzo RA. Comparison of thermogenic effect of fructose and glucose in normal humans. Am J Physiol. 1986 Jun;250(6 Pt 1):E718-24. PubMed PMID: 3521319.

[108] Tappy L, Jéquier E. Fructose and dietary thermogenesis. Am J Clin Nutr. 1993 Nov;58(5 Suppl):766S-770S. doi: 10.1093/ajcn/58.5.766S. Review. PubMed PMID: 8213608.

[109] Simonson DC, Tappy L, Jequier E, Felber JP, DeFronzo RA. Normalization of carbohydrate-induced thermogenesis by fructose in insulin-resistant states. Am J Physiol. 1988 Feb;254(2 Pt 1):E201-7. PubMed PMID: 3279802.

[110] Blaak EE, Saris WH. Postprandial thermogenesis and substrate utilization after ingestion of different dietary carbohydrates. Metabolism. 1996 Oct;45(10): 1235-42. PubMed PMID: 8843178.

[111] Hendler RG, Walesky M, Sherwin RS. Sucrose substitution in prevention and reversal of the fall in metabolic rate accompanying hypocaloric diets. Am J Med. 1986 Aug;81(2):280-4. PubMed PMID: 3740086.

Women fed a high sucrose diet (43% energy) with 71% energy as carbohydrate for 6 weeks had decreases in weight, blood pressure, percentage body fat, depression, hunger and negative mood, with increases in vigilance and positive mood." Results showed that a high sucrose content in a hypoenergetic, low-fat diet did not adversely affect weight loss, metabolism, plasma lipids, or emotional affect."[112]

Fructose intake stimulates the release of GLP1.[113] GLP1 has anti-inflammatory effects that alleviate gut inflammation and improve inflammatory conditions.[114, 115]

---

[112] Surwit RS, Feinglos MN, McCaskill CC, Clay SL, Babyak MA, Brownlow BS, Plaisted CS, Lin PH. Metabolic and behavioral effects of a high-sucrose diet during weight loss. Am J Clin Nutr. 1997 Apr;65(4):908-15. PubMed PMID: 9094871. <https://academic.oup.com/ajcn/article/65/4/908/4655511>

[113] Kuhre RE, Gribble FM, Hartmann B, et al. Fructose stimulates GLP-1 but not GIP secretion in mice, rats, and humans. *Am J Physiol Gastrointest Liver Physiol*. 2014;306(7):G622–G630. doi:10.1152/ajpgi.00372.2013. <https://www.ncbi.nlm.nih.gov/pmc/articles/PMC3962593/>

[114] Anbazhagan AN, Thaqi M, Priyamvada S, et al. GLP-1 nanomedicine alleviates gut inflammation. *Nanomedicine*. 2017;13(2):659–665. doi:10.1016/j.nano.2016.08.004

[115] Hogan AE, Tobin AM, Ahern T, et al. Glucagon-like peptide-1 (GLP-1) and the regulation of human invariant natural killer T cells: lessons from obesity, diabetes and psoriasis. *Diabetologia*. 2011;54(11):2745–2754. doi:10.1007/s00125-011-2232-3. <https://www.ncbi.nlm.nih.gov/pmc/articles/PMC3188710/>

Fructose ingestion may improve mineral status by increasing absorption of magnesium and excretion of phosphorus.[116] Healthy males had significantly more positive balances for copper, zinc, calcium, magnesium and iron when fed a low copper diet providing 20% energy from fructose, compared to a similar diet providing 20% energy from cornstarch.[117]

A fructose diet had no adverse effect on bone quantity or quality.[118] When animals are given a diet with no vitamin D that is 68% sucrose (50:50 fructose:glucose) they have normal blood calcium and bone development, whereas if starch is substituted for sucrose they have low blood and bone calcium.[119]

---

[116] Milne DB, Nielsen FH. The interaction between dietary fructose and magnesium adversely affects macromineral homeostasis in men. J Am Coll Nutr. 2000 Feb;19(1):31-7. PubMed PMID: 10682873. <https://www.ncbi.nlm.nih.gov/pubmed/10682873>

[117] Holbrook JT, Smith JC, Reiser S. Dietary fructose or starch: effects on copper, zinc, iron, manganese, calcium and magnesium balances in humans. Am J Clin Nutr 1989 June;49(6):1290-4. <https://academic.oup.com/ajcn/article-abstract/49/6/1290/4651041?redirectedFrom=fulltext>

[118] Jatkar A, Kurland IJ, Judex S. Diets High in Fat or Fructose Differentially Modulate Bone Health and Lipid Metabolism. *Calcif Tissue Int*. 2017;100(1):20–28. doi:10.1007/s00223-016-0205-8. <https://www.ncbi.nlm.nih.gov/pmc/articles/PMC5217484/>

[119] Artus M. [Effects of administering diets with starch or sucrose basis on certain parameters of calcium metabolism in the young, growing rat]. Ann Nutr Aliment 1975;29(4):305-12.

In fact, fructose makes up 99% of the reducing sugar present in semen. Diminished levels of fructose have been shown to parallel androgen deficiency and the testosterone level.[120] The sperm that won the race to the egg was fueled by fructose, and hence you are here to read about it!

What About Grains?

By now, most people have heard the advice to 'eat more whole grains.' Yet the alleged benefits of consuming whole grains is only in contrast to refined grains. While whole grains do contain nutrients, refined grains are stripped of nutrients during the milling process.

As you will read in Chapter 3, grains are on the Tier 3 list of foods. Tier 3 foods are those foods which we recommend either avoiding, or keeping to a minimum. So why do we relegate grains, including whole grains to the Tier 3 list of foods? A few reasons include:

- Grains contain antinutrients that inhibit absorption of important minerals, including iron and zinc.
- Grains break down into glucose. Fruits and honey provide the ideal ratio of fructose and glucose. Consumption of glucose, in the absence of

---

[120] LabCE, Frutose, https://www.labce.com/spg27422_question.aspx

adequate fructose, or even sucrose impairs blood sugar control because fructose is needed for maximizing liver glycogen storage.
- Unlike fruits, grains lack important polyphenols and bioflavonoids, and are low in potassium, high in phosphorous. Therefore grains are not a good complement to high phosphorus meats, eggs and dairy products.
- Grains are seeds of grasses. Our digestive tracts are not ideally suited for consumption of grasses or their seeds. In order to make grains more digestible, soaking and appropriate cooking methods are required.
- The high fiber and resistant starch content of whole grains can promote excessive gut bacteria growth and stool size, leading to bloating and either constipation (and damage to the rectum and anus) or diarrhea (due to excessive gut acid production by gut bacteria).
- They are an inferior source of protein compared to meats, dairy, and eggs.

All of these concerns equally apply to legumes (beans, peas, lentils). Each person will have to determine whether to include whole or refined grains, (or beans and legumes) into the diet, and at what quantities. Having a bowl of steel cut oats, or split pea soup on a cold winter day may be nostalgic for some. Enjoy it if tolerated. Possibly moderate the total quantity at a meal, or number of days consumed in a week, especially in relation to other grain-based foods, including breads and pastas. As already stated, the dose makes the poison.

In lieu of grains and grain products, we recommend botanical fruits, including winter squashes (butternut, spaghetti, kabocha, acorn, etc.), root vegetables and tubers. Potatoes and root vegetables grow underground, and therefore have lower levels of potential toxins and antinutrients compared to grains and other vegetables, which will be better understood after reading the next section.

What About Vegetables?

Many plants defend themselves from predators by producing toxic chemicals, which are natural pesticides. The above-ground portions of plants are most exposed to predation by animals, so the leaves, stems and seeds (including grains, beans, and nuts) of plants contain the highest levels of these chemicals.

Non-food plants are among the most commonly ingested poisons for children under 5 years of age. However, most people do not know that food plants also contain poisonous compounds. Unfortunately, not many of these have been properly tested for health effects in humans.

Plants produce more of these poisons when under stresses such as high UV light, low temperatures, insect attack, pathogen infection, and nutrient deficiency.[121] Organic food production systems increase the pest and pathogen stress on plants, resulting in increased levels of these toxins in plants.[122] Whole grains provide more of these toxins than refined grains, typical whole grain intakes providing at least several hundred milligrams daily.

When tested in test tubes, many of these chemicals interfere with oxidation reactions, so they can also be called antioxidants. However, the fact that these chemicals behave as antioxidants in test tubes does not prove that they function likewise in the body. In fact it appears that some test-tube phytochemical antioxidants – including vitamin C – are pro-oxidative when in the body.[123] Consequently, it becomes difficult to support claims that the supposed benefits of these phytochemicals stem from their antioxidant effects.

---

[121] Young JE, Zhao X, Carey EE, et al.. Phytochemical phenolics in organically grown vegetables. Mol Nutr Food Res 2005;49:1136-1142.

[122] Baranski M, Srednicka-Tober D, Volakakis N, et al.. Higher antioxidant and low cadmium concentrations and lower incidence of pesticide residues in organically grown crops: a systematic literature review and meta-analysis. Br J Nutr 2014;112:794-811.

[123] Yin J-J, Fu PP, Lutterodt H, Zhou Y-T, Antholine WE, Wamer W. Dual Role of Selected Antioxidants Found in Dietary Supplements: Crossover between Anti- and Pro-oxidant Activities in the Presence of Copper. *Journal of agricultural and food chemistry*. 2012;60(10):2554-2561. doi:10.1021/jf204724w. <https://www.ncbi.nlm.nih.gov/pmc/articles/PMC3971523/>

Evidently, these "antioxidants" function as pesticides and antibiotics. They repel and kill pests and pathogens by poisoning cells, especially nerve cells.

Life depends on oxidation reactions. Oxidation reactions are essential to cellular metabolism. Our cells derive energy from fats through a series of reactions called beta-oxidation. We take in oxygen from the atmosphere to support oxidation of fats and other chemicals, without which we would die. Oxidation reactions can produce loose reactive oxygen species – commonly known as *free radicals* – that could cause collateral damage if not controlled.

Children almost universally reject vegetables because they can taste these bitter poisons (they have more bitter taste receptors than adults to protect them from these toxins) and have not yet been sufficiently programmed to erroneously believe that they need to eat vegetables.

In sufficient quantity, these bitter compounds can poison our digestive system, causing cramping, bloating, diarrhea (as the body attempts to rapidly expel the poison) or constipation (when the gut nerves are paralyzed by a sufficient quantity of the toxins).

Moreover, most vegetables primarily consist of the indigestible carbohydrates collectively called fiber, which has no nutritional benefit but reduces your absorption of essential nutrients causing them to be wasted in your defecation. Leaves, stems, bulbs, flowers, and other fibrous vegetables typically provide less energy than one expends in acquiring them.

The allegedly anti-cancer chemicals naturally occurring in plants are no different. A review[60] of these chemicals gives some interesting information such as:

- Phenols from tea have "cell-killing activity" and inhibit new blood vessel formation.
- High doses of sulforophane from cruciferous vegetables have been shown to induce oxidative stress and cause cell death.

About 99.99% of the pesticides in the typical American diet are phytochemicals that plants use to defend themselves.[124] Americans eat an estimated 1.5 g of natural pesticides daily, which is about 10,000 times more than they eat of synthetic pesticide residues. This includes 5,000 to 10,000 different natural pesticides and their breakdown products.

---

[124] Ames BN, Profet M, Gold LS. Dietary pesticides (99.99% all natural). Proc Natl Acad Sci USA 1990 Oct;87:7777-7781.

For example, cabbage contains at least 49 different natural pesticides and metabolites (Table 1.2).

Table 1.2 Forty-nine natural pesticides and metabolites found in cabbage

Glucosinolates	2-propenyl glucoinolate (sinagrin), 2-methylthiopropyl glucosinolate, 33-methylsulfinylpropyl glucosinolate, 2-butenyl glucosinolate, 2-hydroxy-3-butenyl glucosinolate, 4-methylthiobutyl glucosinolate, 4-methysuflinylbutyl glucosinolate, 4-methylsulfonylbutyl glucosinolate, beyzyl glucosinolate, 2-phenylethyl glucosinolate, propyl glucosinolate, butyl glucosinolate
Indole glucosinolates and related indoles	3-indolylmethyl glucosinolate (glucobrassicin), 1-methoxy-3-indolylmethyl glocosinolate (neoglucobrassicin), indole-3-carbinol, indole-3-acetonitrile, bis(3-indolyl)methane
Isothiocyanates and goitrin	allyl isothiocyanate, 3-methylthiopropyl isothiocyanate, 3-methylsulfinylpropyl isothiocyanate, 3-butenyl isothiocyanate, 5-vinyloxazolidine-2-thione (goitrin), 4-methylthiobutyl isothiocyanate, 4-methylsulfinylbutyl isothiocyanate, 4-methylsulfonylbutyle isothiocyanate, 4-pentenyl isothiocyanate, benzyl isotyocyanate, phenylethyl isothyocyanate
Cyanides	1-cyano-2,3-epithiopropane, 1-cyano-3,4-epithiobutane, 1-cyano-3,4-epithiopentane, *threo*-1-cyano-2-hydroxy-3,4-epithiobutane, *erythro*-1-cyano-2-hydroxy-3,4-epithiobutane, 2-phenylpropionitrile, allyl cyanide, 1-cyano-2-hydroxy-3-butene, 1-cyano-3-methylsulfinylpropane, 1-cyano-4-methylsuflinylbutane
Terpenes	menthol, neomenthol, isomenthol, carvone
Phenols	2-methoxyphenol, 3-caffoylquinic acid (chlorogenic acid), 4-caffoylquinic acid, 5-caffoylqunic acid (neochlorogenic acid), 4-(*p*-coumaroyl)quniic acid, 5-(p-coumaroyl)quinic acid, 5-feruloylquinic acid

Source: Ames BN, Profet M, Gold LS. Dietary pesticides (99.99% all natural). Proc Natl Acad Sci USA 1990 Oct;87:7777-7781.

Some of the phytochemicals which have been touted as anti-cancer anti-oxidants have also been proven to be mutagenic and carcinogenic in the same type of animal studies used to test safety of man-made pesticides. Researchers have only tested 53 naturally occurring plant pesticides for carcinogenicity, but 27 have tested positive. These rodent carcinogens naturally occur in: anise, apple, apricot, banana, basil, broccoli, Brussels sprouts, cabbage, cantaloupe, caraway, carrot, cauliflower, celery, cherries, cinnamon, cloves, cocoa, coffee, collard greens, comfrey herb tea, currants, dill, eggplant, endive, fennel, grapefruit juice, grapes, guava, honey, honeydew melon, horseradish, kale, lentils, lettuce, mango, mushrooms, mustard, nutmeg, orange juice, parsley, parsnip, peach, pear, peas, black pepper, pineapple, plum, potato, radish, raspberries, rosemary, sesame seeds, tarragon, tea, tomato, and turnip. Probably every fruit and vegetable in the supermarket contains natural plant pesticides that are rodent carcinogens, at concentrations that are thousands of times higher than the levels of synthetic pesticides allowed on foods.[125]

---

[125] Ames BN, Profet M, Gold LS. Dietary pesticides (99.99% all natural). Proc Natl Acad Sci USA 1990 Oct;87:7777-7781.

At least 72 of these natural plant pesticides have been shown to be clastogenic – capable of breaking chromosomes – in at least one test, at doses far less than they naturally occur in foods. For example, allyl isothiocyanate exhibited clastogenicity at 0.0005 ppm, which is about 200,000 times less than the concentration of sinigrin, its glucosinolate, in cabbage. Caffeic acid proved clastogenic at a concentration of 260 and 500 ppm, which is less than its concentration in roasted coffee beans and close to its concentration in apples, lettuce, endive, and potato skin. Chlorogenic acid, a precursor of caffeic acid, proved clastogenic at a concentration of 150 ppm, which is 100 times less than its concentration in roasted coffee beans and similar to its concentration in apples, pears, plums, peaches, cherries, and apricots.[126] Chlorogenic acid and caffeic acid are also mutagens.

In plants, these compounds occur in measures of parts per thousand or million, whereas synthetic pesticide residues generally occur in parts per billion. Whereas you may be able to wash man-made pesticides off of foods, you can't wash naturally occurring pesticides out of foods.

---

[126] Ibid.

Many parts of plants taste quite bitter from high concentrations of these chemicals. Just the bitter flavor will repel many predators, but if it doesn't, the bitter stuff may injure or even kill healthy cells or tissues.

Remember, mutations and cancer are only the extreme effects of exposure to large amounts these chemicals. Any chemical that in high doses alters cell function enough to cause mutations or initiate tumors very likely will in smaller doses cause less severe disorders of cell function.

For example the goitrins in plants interfere with iodine metabolism, and about 8 million people world-wide have goiter and hypothyroidism because they consume goitrin-rich diets in combination with insufficient iodine.[127] Plant foods that have some constituents with goitrogenic activity include:

- Vegetables: Arugula, asparagus, bok choy, broccoli, broccolini, Brussels sprouts, cabbage, cauliflower, Chinese broccoli, Chinese cabbage, choy sum, collard greens, kale, kohlrabi, mizuna, mustard greens, onions, parsley, radishes, rapini, rutabagas, spinach, turnips, wasabi, watercress
- Roots and tubers: Cassava, horseradish, sweet potato
- Grains: Millet, corn

---

[127] Whitney EN and Rolfes SR. Understanding Nutrition 10th Edition. Thomson Wadsworth, 2005:451.

- Seeds: Flax, canola, mustard
- Legumes: Soybeans, soy products, peanuts, lima beans
- Fruits: Apples, apricots, blueberries, citrus fruits, cranberries, grapes, peaches, strawberries

Of these, the cabbage family vegetables, cassava, millet, seeds and legumes have the most potent antithyroid activity when they form a large part of the diet and dietary iodine is limited. People who avoid eating animal products have a much higher risk of iodine deficiency than people who eat animal products. One study reported that one-fourth of vegetarians and 80 percent of vegans suffer from iodine deficiency compared to only 9 percent of meat-eaters.[128]

---

[128] Kajcovincová-Kudlácková M, Bucková K, Klimes I, Seboková E. Iodine deficiency in vegetarians and vegans. Ann Nutr Metab 2003;47(5):183-5.

Compared to omnivores and carnivores, vegetarians and others who emphasize eating whole plant foods will consume greater amounts of all plant toxins including goitrogens. Some research indicates a higher incidence of cancer, allergies, and mental health disorders, a higher need and use of health care services, and a poorer quality of life for vegetarians, despite their mean lower body mass index, higher mean socioeconomic status, and better health behavior including greater physical activity and less use of alcohol and tobacco.[129]

Plants produce sweet fruits to entice and reward animals for dispersing their seeds, creating a win-win symbiotic relationship with the animals that eat the fruits. If fruits poisoned the animals that eat them, animals would be discouraged from helping the plant distribute its seeds. Further, animals that can tolerate or even make use of the mild toxins in fruits can also gain the nutritional benefits of the nutrients in those fruits. As already mentioned it appears we are among the animals so equipped, because we have salivary proline-rich proteins that neutralize the alleged anti-nutrient polyphenol flavonoids (tannins) which are the principal "toxins" found in fruits.

---

[129] Burkert NT, Muckenhuber J, Grobschadl F, et al.. Nutrition and Health – The Association between Eating Behavior and Various Health Parameters: A Matched Sample Study. PLoS One 9(2):e88278. doi:10.1371/journal.pone.0088278

Compared to leaves, stems and seeds, roots and tubers generally have lower toxin levels because they are protected from predation by their location underground. Carrots may be particularly valuable because they have have antimicrobial activity which may help kill harmful intestinal bacteria that produce endotoxin.[130] Also, the fiber in carrots binds with endotoxin to carry it out of the gut.

Since the dose makes the poison, with the **HIGH VITALITY DIET** we aim to reduce our exposure to plant toxins by generally limiting or avoiding the parts of plants with the highest levels of potentially harmful toxins: leaves, stems, seeds, nuts, grains and legumes.

However, it is also possible to over-consume fruits, particularly highly acid fruits. Excessive intake of sugars and acidic fruits can cause tooth erosion and decay. As true for every nutrient, there exists a sweet spot where you get benefits without harms, below which you may suffer harm from deficiency and above which you may suffer harm from excess.

---

[130] Babic I, Nguyen-the C, Amiot MJ, Aubert S. Antimicrobial activity of shredded carrot extracts on food-borne bacteria and yeast. J Appl Microbiology 1994 Feb;76(2):135-141. <https://onlinelibrary.wiley.com/doi/abs/10.1111/j.1365-2672.1994.tb01608.x>

In summary, **MEATS & SWEETS ~ A HIGH VITALITY DIET** is not an authoritarian approach. Animal foods, including muscle meats, eggs, dairy foods, and gelatin plus glycine supplementation added to beverages, or made into jello, and/or gelatinous-rich parts of animals provide essential nutrients in the most bioavailable form, while fruits and honey ~ the sweets ~ are ideal complements to the more energy dense animal foods.

Many people choose foods based on isolated information about each food, often instigated by dietary faddism. Optimizing your genetic potential for health is more about achieving the right balance of macro and micro-nutrients, as too little, or too much of meats *or* sweets can detract from rather than support and enhance both physical and mental health. Getting adequate intake of important macro- and micronutrients including folate choline, B vitamins, calcium, magnesium, iron, zinc, polyphenols, and bio-flavonoids can help prevent premature aging, with physical degeneration and cognitive decline ~ now prevalent among our aging population.

3 - THE 3 TIERS OF FOODS

As mentioned in the previous chapters, every plant or animal food has potentially toxic side effects if continually consumed in excess, while too little creates deficiencies. Keep in mind, nothing is acting in isolation. Constituents of foods are best optimized in the right ratio with other nutrients.

A miraculous symphony of events transpires that result in our being alive, and able to live a high vitality life. Your body desires peak functioning! Each person must learn to trust their true nature, apply reasoning, and experiment to determine what combination and quantities of meats and sweets, or total protein, fats, and carbs will be best tolerated to best thrive.

Supplementation of herbs, vitamins, minerals, enzymes, or glandulars may be necessary to restore optimal health of the digestive system, thyroid, and other systems. For example, magnesium deficiency is common among Americans. Magnesium deficiency can be due to inadequate intake, poor absorption, or increased secretion due to alcoholism, diuretics, kidney disease, oral contraceptive use, and too high calcium. Low levels of magnesium can lead to an increased susceptibility to a variety of diseases, including:

- heart disease
- high blood pressure (HBP)
- kidney stones
- cancer
- insomnia
- PMS + menstrual cramping
- irritability
- weakness
- heart disturbances
- problems with nerve conduction and muscle contraction
- muscle cramps
- loss of appetite
- predisposition to stress, anxiety and depression

Magnesium supplementation can potentially benefit several conditions including: asthma, cardiovascular disease, angina, HBP, stroke, diabetes, hearing loss, fatigue, hypoglycemia, kidney stones, migraines, osteoporosis, PMS, glaucoma and more.[131]

Meats & Sweets are prioritized according to 3 tiers, as follows:

- **Tier 1 foods** are the most nutrient rich foods which research supports to be the best for supporting healthy functioning of the body. These are foods to base the bulk of your diet around. Especially include dairy foods if tolerated for calcium, eggs,

---

[131] Encyclopedia of Nutritional Supplements, Prima Publishing, 1996, Michael T. Murray

and fruits including fresh orange juice, Concord grape juice, jello or collagen supplementation, and a raw carrot or carrot salad each or most days between or before your main meal.
- **Tier 2 foods** are either a little less beneficial, and/or those foods which are complementary to Tier 1 foods that you would naturally eat a smaller quantity of, such as cooking fats and alternative sweeteners.
- **Tier 3 foods** include those foods that should either be greatly minimized, or totally avoided. Tier 3 foods tend to be the most potentially damaging to health. Eliminating the unhealthy PUFA oils and hydrogenated fats is especially critical.

Tier 1 Foods

- **Dairy** - milk, yogurt, and cheese, including ricotta cheese (fresh is best!) & cottage cheese from cow, sheep, goat, etc. (low-fat or whole)
- **Juice** - orange juice (fresh squeezed is usually best) & Concord grape juice
- **Fruit** - seasonal, fresh or frozen, stewed, poached, baked & dried fruits
- **Eggs**
- **Gelatin and collagen-rich, gelatinous foods** - fruit or milk jello, collagen & powdered glycine added to liquids, &/or bone broths, soups, or stews made with joints and glycine-rich parts of animals, such as oxtail, shank bones, & chicken feet

- **Meats** - lean cuts of meat, prioritizing beef, wild game, wild turkey, mutton, lamb or other meats local to your region
- **Liver** (aim for 2 oz. 2-3 x per week) or other organ meats ~ you may substitute powdered liver mixed with a vegetable juice if needed
- **Fish** - mild white fish like cod, sole, perch, trout; Keta salmon
- **Shellfish** - ideally sustainably harvested shrimp, clams, mussels, crab; fresh or smoked canned oysters in extra virgin olive oil (XVOO)
- **Carrots** - 1 daily raw carrot or Carrot Salad
- **Botanical fruits** - (fruits commonly referred to as vegetables) cucumbers, summer squash
- **Fungi** - mushrooms (all varieties)
- **Vegetables** - onions, garlic, fresh herbs; carrots & celery for cooking soups, soft field green or wild lettuces - all only as desired & tolerated
- **Beverages** -water, coffee, tea, fruit flavored mineral water, ketone drinks
- **Sweets** - honey -ideally raw or local, real maple syrup and other tree saps

Tier 2 Foods

- **Dairy** - cream, half & half, butter
- **Juice** - cranberry juice, fresh apple juice or cider, &/or other fresh or jarred juices for making jello ~ preferring juices without preservatives, coloring, added sugars

- **Fruit** - organic/better quality canned fruit in natural juices
- **Meats** - fattier cuts of meat; poultry, pork, etc.
- **Fish** - wild salmon, sardines or mackerel packed in extra virgin olive oil (XVOO), water, or tomato sauce (not in other commercial plant or seed oils), other fish with low mercury count
- **Botanical fruits** - winter squashes, tomatoes, peppers (tomatoes and bell peppers may trigger joint pain for some), olives and avocados
- **Vegetables** - cabbages ~ naturally brined and/or cooked, salad greens, beet greens, organic or local potatoes & fingerlings & other tubers & root veggies including rutabaga, beet roots, turnips, etc. (sweet potatoes are higher in oxalate acids ~ consume at your discretion)
- **Beverages** - wine, hard ciders, beer if tolerated ~ all in moderation
- **Sweets** - organic sugars, coconut sugar, molasses, monk fruit, stevia, Xyla, Swerve, cane or brown sugar, etc.; ice cream made as naturally and simply as able to find or make your own! (Haagen Das vanilla, strawberry, chocolate, pineapple coconut and a couple others have the fewest ingredients); better quality cheesecake, 85%+ dark chocolate
- **Fats** - coconut meat, milk, or oil, MCT oil, or sustainably harvested palm oil, butter or ghee, and extra virgin olive oil (XVOO) are the best choices, other saturated fats from animals or fruit oils include tallow, avocado oil, or occasional nut oils (pecan, macadamia, hazelnut) for flavoring

- **Seasonings** - salt, and other seasonings, fresh and/or dried herbs, seaweed, small amounts of vinegar

Tier 3 Foods

- **Hydrogenated and partially hydrogenated oils** ~ fats labeled *partially hydrogenated* or *hydrogenated* including palm, cottonseed, or corn oil should be avoided
- **Polyunsaturated Oils** - also known as PUFAs ~ commercially refined oils from fish, plants and seeds, including cod liver, corn, soy, sunflower, sesame seed and canola oils, and other commercial plant oils (and vegan butters) are pro-inflammatory, and impair the body's ability to appropriately metabolize sugar, possibly leading to insulin resistance and diabetes, among many other health issues, hence should be avoided
- **Sweeteners** - synthetic sweeteners and refined sugars, including saccharin, aspartame, acesulfame, neotame, and sucralose ~ sweeteners that go by the brand names of *Equal* or *Sweet and Low* should be avoided
- **Nuts & seeds** - including the now popular flax and chia seeds, along with most other seeds and most nuts should generally be avoided, or consumed minimally; nuts lower in PUFA fats, and higher in saturated fats, such as pecans, macadamia nuts, or hazelnuts, and possibly walnuts may be enjoyed if tolerated in small amounts

- **Grains** - whole grains including oatmeal, brown rice, quinoa, millet, etc., and refined grain products, including white rice, bulgur, couscous, grits, breads, muffins, pastas, crackers, cookies, pretzels, scones, waffles, pancakes, etc. are best kept to a minimum; some may need to totally avoid all grains, and other gluten containing foods to restore health
- **Snacks** - dry crunchy snack foods should be kept to a minimum and those with the PUFA oils should be avoided
- **Additives** - guar gums, and other food thickeners, additives, food dyes, and preservatives should be avoided as much as possible
- **GMOs** - avoid genetically modified foods as much as possible

Food Selection Guidelines

- Make the bulk of your food selections from the Tier 1 food list.
- Supplement as you *desire*, and as you believe you can *well tolerate* foods from Tier 2 ~ however, do not feel obligated.
- Consume Tier 3 foods as needed, whether while traveling, visiting family or friends, dining out, or because you just are really craving an old familiar favorite food. Whether indulging, or celebrating, do so without guilt. Just choose consciously, and enjoy! However it's best to avoid PUFA oils and hydrogenated fats ~ as much as able!

- Adjust how you 'stack' your meals ~ the order in which you eat meats and sweets ~ and quantities of each until you find your sweet spot!
- If you have avoided fruits and sugars for some time, or have been on any type of restrictive or low-carbohydrate diet, add fruit and honey back slowly. Try having fruit as your first meal ~ alone, or with yogurt and honey, eggs, coffee or a latte, or as a snack or appetizer before a meal.
- If craving starchy foods, or lacking in fruit options, substitute the best juices possible, dried fruit, winter squashes when in season, or tubers.
- Supplement with enzymes, herbs, or vitamins and minerals as needed, and as prescribed by your health care provider. Also see Resources at the end.
- Practice trusting the cravings of your body over your mind. Learning to trust your true nature is a practice, and takes time.
- Don't over analyze every symptom, automatically associating each symptom with a particular food, or even the last food consumed. What you think is a trigger for a symptom may not be!
- Remember with all foods, *the dose makes the poison*. A food can be highly beneficial for you at one dose, but not at another. How much total protein, fat, and fruit or carbs in general you tolerate will vary over time, and from others. Go by what works best for you, not others.
- It is common to experience mild digestive upset including bloating or change of stools when

making changes to one's diet. Ride the tide, as better health is at hand.

Some foods will be more or less tolerated, depending on one's current condition, and particular constitution. The ideal to keep in mind is to choose to eat in a manner that will help you best thrive, and that will support you on a hormonal, biological, metabolic and cellular level.

Instead of focusing solely on immediate results, or changes to your body weight, tune within, and pay attention to subtle changes. Note if your moods feel more calm, if you sleep better, if you have less joint pain, your skin looks healthier, or other changes. Have patience as you let your body do what it needs once given the right raw materials. Similarly, if having a 'craving' for example, pause before making a choice. Ask yourself, *'What am I really needing right now? Some protein? Fruit or something sweet? Maybe I am a bit stressed, and a little sugar will help! Am I even hungry, or just grabbing something to avoid facing my true feelings?'*

One benefit of our **MEATS & SWEETS** dietary approach is how simple it can be! Fill up on milk ~ which you can sweeten if you desire ~ or milk products, such as cheese, cottage cheese, ricotta cheese, yogurt ~ along with some eggs, fruits, and whatever types of lean meats, poultry, fish, and shellfish you feel most drawn to. And yes, sometimes a bowl of ice cream before bed, or a healthy made cheesecake for breakfast can be precisely what the doctor ordered!

Be sure to include gelatinous-rich cuts, such as chicken feet, ox tail, or shank bones, cooked into bone broth or stews. If you have no inkling to prepare these cuts of meat ~ and even if you do ~ consider regular consumption of supplemental beef collagen and glycine stirred into drinks, or made into jello. (To order, see the Resources chapter at the end.)

What About Weight Loss?

There is a lot that can be written about the mechanisms of weight loss, the details of which many promoting very low-carb or ketogenic diets seem to either be unaware of or over look. As mentioned in the introduction, we encourage focusing on improving one's metabolic health. That includes supporting the health of the thyroid and adrenals, and eating to boost one's metabolism, rather than suppress it ~ which is what happens when people are fasting, or eating only one meal per day. It is vitally important to minimize cortisol production which can be accomplished in part from our meats and sweets dietary approach, and finding ways to reduce stress through appropriate lifestyle choices. Hi stress plus poor sleep will impede weight loss.

It is not uncommon for people who commence a high-fat, low-carb or ketogenic diet to lose weight seemingly effortlessly initially. Some of this is the loss of glycogen reserves and water. Encouraged, many continue. After some time, the fat loss plateaus. Many then switch to a higher protein Carnivore or Zero Carb diet, still keeping carbohydrate consumption low.

Common complaints of folks who continue on low-carb diets, whether higher in protein, fat, or both include:

- Muscle cramping, especially at night
- Increased irritability or easier to get angry or frustrated
- Fat weight loss stalls, or comes back on
- Increased cravings for sweets
- Hair may be falling out in more noticeable clumps
- Appetite between meals lessens, able to go longer between meals (while a seemingly good sign, it can also indicate a slowed metabolism)
- Increased cholesterol
- Drowsy post meals
- Feelings of failure to thrive, or recover from training

The energy producing processes in your body will preferentially choose to burn sugar for fuel when given the opportunity. The belief in ketogenic and carnivore diet circles is that if you are consuming very little carbohydrate it will cause your body to burn your own body fat for fuel. Many begin to eat only one meal a day, or practice intermittent fasting to aid in the body's ability to burn it's own fat for fuel, yet may unwittingly be triggering a stress response by both fasting and insufficient intake of sugar!

In the distant past, if humans went for extended periods of time without much available food, the forced fasting would cause the body to increase cortisol production. This triggered a chemical chain of events, leading to the body metabolizing it's own protein and fat stores for fuel. This process aided in our survival, yet it isn't an ideal state to intentionally mimic in modern times. If cortisol is being released, it's like sending out an emergency alert to the rest of the body. Cortisol is elevated during times of stress and duress, and contributes greatly to fat storage, weight gain, lowered immunity, premature aging, and a myriad of other concerns.

We have sweet taste receptors on our tongue for a reason. Unfortunately, many people believe they lack will power when craving sweets, yet the body has these powerful cravings because it is begging for sugar. The right kind of sugar. Fructose!

MEATS & SWEETS ~ A HIGH VITALITY DIET is designed to give your body what it needs to function at *peak* efficiency. While everyone wants fast results with respect to weight loss, this may not be healthy, especially long term. Neither will it help you realize your optimal blueprint for thriving health.

Excess consumption of fat much above thirty to possibly forty percent of total calories, give or take, may impede your body's ability to use, or oxidize sugar for energy. Even if 'forced' to burn fat for energy, the process is not optimal. Any amount of fat consumed above what the body will metabolize for energy will store as fat.

According to Ray Peat and many others, when you consume a diet high in milk, juice, fruit, and some eggs, meats, and shellfish ~ meats & sweets ~ with low to modest amount of added fats, minimal to no grains and beans, and only the minimal amount of PUFA fats found in some meats, ideally below 10 g daily, the body will eventually lose excess fat weight at a very slow but safe rate, without raising cortisol levels.

Said in another way, when you eat the foods that naturally keep cortisol levels to a minimum, and that will aid in the insulin's ability to do it's job effectively, your hormones will function better, your nerves will be more calm, and you are less likely to feel as though you are living in an ongoing, sub level state of flight or fight.

The thyroid gland produces thyroxine (T4) and the liver converts T4 to triiodothyronine (T3). To make the conversion, the liver needs adequate carbohydrate. The thyroid controls metabolism and thermoregulation in the body. When your thyroid is healthy, your metabolism will also be healthy, and you will be more adaptable to temperature changes.

Hypothyroidism is when the thyroid gland under produces thyroid hormones, leading to a slowing down effect. Primary symptoms of an under functioning thyroid include:

- Sluggish metabolism
- Weight gain that is difficult to lose
- Cold hands and feet
- Sensitive to cold
- Sluggish or fatigued
- Difficult to get going in the morning
- Body doesn't perspire easily
- Possible increased depression or anxiety

Hyperthyroidism is an over production of thyroid hormones, leading to the opposite symptoms, including:

- Sudden weight loss, with difficult time gaining
- Sensitivity to heat, or sweat a lot
- Possible increased irritability or anxiousness

What many people may not understand about thyroid health is that it is part of a loop, or axis that includes the pituitary, liver and adrenals. A patient may present symptoms of fatigue, sluggish metabolism and weight gain to a medical doctor, who will test for low thyroid hormones. If low, they will prescribe a synthetic thyroid. However, it may come back in the 'normal' range. This could be a result of a malfunctioning somewhere else on the axis, such as poor liver conversion, adrenal hormone production, or even poor functioning of the pituitary gland, which is the primary gland that communicates with the thyroid to stimulate thyroid hormone production.

Of course, another reason that someone can present low thyroid symptoms, but test normal is because what Western medicine has deemed a 'normal' range may not reflect an 'optimal' range. We believe what you and most people prefer is what is *optimal*, not just *normal*.

One more piece to the fat loss puzzle that is now being considered more prominently in research studies is the role of gut flora in nutrient absorption and overall health. **MEATS & SWEETS ~ A HIGH VITALITY DIET** aims to minimize endotoxin production in and absorption from the gut. Endotoxins are produced when eating high-fiber diets, especially fibers from grains and beans. Orange and Concord grape juices help *prevent* endotoxin absorption. Daily Carrot Salad consumption helps kill harmful bacteria and provides pectin fiber to carry endotoxin out of the gut, helping maintain a healthier gut microbiome. Yogurt also reduces endotoxin absorption. Mushrooms in larger quantities may work as well.

If you are experiencing a lot of bloating from increased consumption of whole fruits, you may try upping the juice, milk, honey or syrup, and reducing the amount of whole fruit, adjusting as your gut health improves. Supplementing with quality digestive enzymes may also be necessary.

Diets higher in meats and non-fruit plant foods, especially beans and whole grains, without dairy foods, can result in disorders due to calcium deficiency and phosphorus excess over time. In order to achieve at least a 1:1 ratio of calcium to phosphorous, dairy is among the staple foods of the **High Vitality Diet**. Most people can tolerate fermented dairy (such as yogurt or kefir). If you don't tolerate dairy we recommend supplementing with calcium. Typically calcium carbonate is optimal as the carbonate itself has metabolic benefits as a precursor to beneficial carbon dioxide. Eggshell calcium is another affordable alternative that is easy to make yourself.

The importance of consuming adequate levels of minerals can't be overstated. Our soils no longer contain the levels of minerals they once did. Excess stress, and even mentally taxing jobs can really burn up energy. Supplementing with minerals may help counteract some of these deficiencies. There is a liquid zinc test you can purchase to determine if zinc deficient. Experiment with taking additional calcium and magnesium, and possibly an additional trace mineral supplement along with digestive enzymes to increase absorption for 3-4 weeks and see if this improves energy, especially when extra stressed out. See Resources section for ordering options.

One final point I would like to emphasize. I suspect that many people, and especially women have been led to believe that filling up on lots of greens and huge salads is essential to maintain regular elimination, or alkalinity. Yet, these foods were never historically consumed in great quantities, as most modern vegetables are hybridized versions of the original plant. As discussed in Chapter 2, there are many components in above ground leaves and stalks ~ modern cultivated greens and vegetables, including organic ~ that could be unwittingly sabotaging your health. Also, when consuming huge bowls of salad, you are filling yourself up with water, non-essential fibers, and low nutrient-dense foods, filling your stomach up without necessarily providing essential nutrients. This can cause bloating, digestive distress, and increased hunger as these bulking foods replace more nutrient rich alternatives.

Don't take my word for it. Consuming some greens and vegetables is far less worrisome than consuming refined grains and PUFA oils. However, if you have conditions that are not resolving, and you consume lots of salads, green smoothies, and other greens and vegetables, it may be a worthwhile experiment to cut way back or even eliminate these foods for 3-4 weeks or more to note if symptoms improve. Also, as previously mentioned, digestive enzymes may be necessary to improve digestion and absorption of important minerals and other essential nutrients.

Trouble Shooting

- Trust your gut! Let your inner divine knowing guide your choices.
- We have many preconceived ideas about food and health. The analytical mind is quick to jump to conclusions about which foods caused which symptoms. Maybe that is correct. Maybe it isn't!
- There are so many nerves in the gut, which is why anxiety and worry can disrupt digestion. Remain open and mindful to what you are feeling when eating. Try to avoid eating while in a hurry or upset when possible.
- If you are super sensitive to all but a narrow range of foods, you have a couple of options: 1) Continue to only eat those narrow ranges of foods if you are content to do so, and it alleviates uncomfortable symptoms, or 2) Dig deeper, and discover what *within you* is needing healing in order to better

tolerate a healthy variety of foods as intended by Nature! It isn't always about the foods. If you want to experience greater freedom, and higher vitality, it may be worth investing time and resources into resolving underlying issues ~ both physical and emotional ~ that can trigger symptoms including unresolved emotional wounds, anger, resentments, anxiety, fear, worry, stress, and/or poor sleep which can negatively impact your health. Supplements, or other therapies may be required.

- You don't need to obsess over eating perfectly clean foods. Perfectionism is a reflection of a hyper need to control one's environment. Instead, try to cultivate beliefs that the food you have is nourishing you on every level. Bless it. Be grateful for it. I know it is popular to expound the virtues of all things pure, clean, pristine, organic, grass-fed and finished, and/or raw. These things are not wrong, unless they prevent you from eating the right foods. Contrary to popular opinion, raw dairy is not always best. Raw meat is not always best. Many more people get sick from raw dairy than commercial dairy, as noted by the U.S. Centers for Disease Control (CDC). Learn to hunt, support local farmers or raise your own food if and when able, by all means. When you can't, bless the abundance of food choices available to feed the masses, and thank the animals, farmers, ranchers, and all others involved in the process of making the food you are eating available for you with relative ease.

- The goal is to enjoy *increasing vitality and a sweet life*, with greater resilience to stress, and any type of environmental, emotional, or dietary triggers. Find ways to *tweak your life, and not just your diet* to keep stress to a minimum! **Some examples:** Live where you can reduce your daily commute, create meaningful work or work from home, get barefoot outdoors to ground or spend time in Nature to recharge, recreate, and get adequate sunshine for absorption of Vitamin D. Find your tribe of like-minded folks who share your values, read spiritual and uplifting books, listen to uplifting or relaxing music, heal old emotional wounds, forgive those who may have harmed you (including your parents) or do what you need to feel whole, integrated, and grateful for life!
- Some folks who follow Ray Peat consume colas or other beverages sweetened with sugar (versus the synthetic sweeteners found in diet drinks.) Real sugar is favorable to synthetic sweeteners, however, we recommend prioritizing whichever combination of fruit, juices, honey, and/or tree saps works best for you, as these foods have more nutritional value than cane sugars.
- Add fruit and honey into your diet **incrementally.** Peel fruit like apples when just beginning, especially if you have been following a very low-carbohydrate or ketogenic diet. Minimize or eliminate grains, beans, and stalky, fibrous vegetables ~ at least long enough to restore gut health.

- As previously mentioned, how you stack your meals can make a difference. By stacking, I mean the order in which you eat certain foods throughout the day. For example, some people prefer to enjoy fruit or a large glass of orange juice first thing in the morning, on an empty stomach. It digests very quickly into useable energy. Others may need to consume fruit with protein and/or fat. Protein provides satiety, but so does fruit! Fruit before meals can help manage total calories consumed at that meal, and alleviate post meal sweets cravings. Fruit with meat can prevent post meal crashes.
- When just beginning to eat more fruits and total carbs after following a low-carbohydrate diet ~ you may experience a sensation of 'rehydrating.' On low-carb diets, the initial weight loss is typically water loss, which is used otherwise to store glycogen. Adding carbohydrates back into the diet will cause the body to do this in reverse. Water will be retained to help replenish glycogen storage. So to the ladies reading this, hang tight if you experience a 'filling out' or bloating at first. I did. It will pass.
- Dried fruit, or fruit and cheese makes for easy to carry snacks.
- Orange or concord grape juices provide many benefits, as previously mentioned, so when in need of some fast fuel, consider having either.
- Another quick and easy source of liquid food is milk! If out at a coffee shop, steamed milk, with or

without coffee or espresso, sweetened with honey or a little raw sugar and/or stevia is a great snack.
- Seaweed is a good source of iodine, which supports thyroid functioning. A one to two inch piece a few days per week should be adequate. Or use a seaweed seasoning blend on food.
- Drink enough liquid, but don't feel like you have to 'pound' down several liters of water each day. Drink to thirst. I believe many women drink more fluid than is able to be processed and filtered by the body, taxing the kidneys. You may want to research this further.
- It may take a little experimenting to find the total percentages of protein, fat, and carbohydrates that suit you the best. I go with my cravings, which some days is for more meats, some days more sweets! I crave more fresh fruit during the summer, more dried fruit, honey, and possibly winter squash (a botanical fruit), or tubers during the winter.
- **Over forty females** may need to have more lean protein, especially to maintain an ideal body mass index, aiming for +/- 100g per day. If experiencing bouts of abdominal fullness and pain, you may need to take some supplements to improve bile flow. Women over forty who have been on really low-fat diets are at higher risk for gallstones.
- **Supplements we recommend:** Artichoke extract, Standard Process Livton, ox bile extract, or digestive enzymes with HCL can help promote healthy bile flow, especially if you have been eating a very low-fat, low animal food diet. Magnesium

can help with muscle cramping, constipation, and improved calcium absorption. Calcium and trace minerals are very important to our overall health, energy, and ability to mitigate stress. Glandulars or herbal supplements like ashwaganda and others can be taken to support the thyroid and adrenal glands and endocrine system. Vitamin K2 supports bone health. Check with your health care provider, and see listings in the Resource section.
- Keep it simple, and choose the best *meat* or *sweet* available, then savor it, and celebrate life! While at a coffee shop, I enjoy steamed milk or a latte. I usually carry dried fruit with me, but if out, I opt for a piece of cheesecake or maybe a coconut macaroon or croissant or over bagels, muffins, cookies, quick breads, and other refined flour products. You may prefer juice, or something else. The key is to do your best. My Mom is from Belgium, so I guess I inherited my penchant for croissants and dark chocolate! I may indulge a couple times per year, and when I do, I ***really*** enjoy it. Warmed, and with more butter on top. I'm talking I *savor every bite*, then I lick my fingers afterwards! *Life is meant to be sweet!*

A word about the recipes

I have always loved cooking, and have worked in catering and the food industry the first half of my life. These days, however, I am the queen of simple! I spent hours of my day shopping, storing, preparing, cooking, and cleaning up when eating a plant-based, macrobiotic diet. Not anymore! Simple meals means more time to enjoy other pursuits in my life, while still preparing 99% of all my food at home!

The recipes that follow are *very* simple. Tweak them as you like, swapping out your favorite protein as desired. I have added alternative protein sources in parentheses in some recipes. Choose what appeals to you.

Experiencing high vitality does not need to be complicated. Eat whole foods, and avoid getting ensnared by societal boxes, so you can enjoy a sweet life!

4 - MEATS
Eggs, Meats, Fish & Bone Broth

Eggs

Who doesn't know how to cook eggs? Eggs are nutrient rich, affordable, simple to prepare, and easy to carry. Rather than include lots of egg recipes, I kept it minimal. I included my often asked for recipe for softly boiled eggs, plus Eggnog, Deviled Eggs, and homemade Mayonnaise, below.

Softly Boiled Eggs

5-6 eggs (I have 2, Don has 3)
Filtered water to cover
Bowl of cold water ~ I keep a bottle of cold water in the fridge just for the eggs as the colder the water, the better

Place eggs in a big enough pot for each egg to have a little space to breathe. Cover with filtered water. Bring to a boil on medium-high heat. For soft boiled eggs that remain a little runny, remove eggs as soon as you see the water begins to come up to boil. You should see bigger bubbles forming, and the movement of the water quickening. Immediately plunge eggs into bowl with enough cold water to cover, then refrigerate. This should help the eggs be able to peel better, but it's not totally foolproof.

If you don't want to deal with peeling the eggs, try what we do. Use a knife to whack the egg in the center, then scoop out each half onto a plate or small bowl. Otherwise, crack with the back of the knife around the edges, peel the top half, and eat eggs out of a shot glass.

If you prefer fully hard boiled, turn the heat lower once it begins to boil. Let simmer a few minutes, then remove as above.

Poached Eggs

Pot filled with 2-3 inches of water, and a steamer basket
A small heatproof metal or ceramic bowl
A little fat ~ butter, olive oil, or a spray
1-2+ eggs per person
Seasoning - salt, pepper, paprika, and/or dried parsley, or granulated dulse
Grated cheese, optional

Heat pot with water on medium-high heat. Meanwhile, wipe (or spray) a little fat of choice inside the bowl. Crack eggs into bowl, and season as desired. Place bowl in steamer basket, in the pot. Cover, turn to medium, and let cook until the whites on top are no longer liquid, trying not to over cook. About 6-8 minutes.

If using grated cheese, add half-way through cooking.

Deviled Eggs

6 eggs, hard boiled
1/4 cup of Mayonnaise (Use mayo made with avocado or olive oil, or make your own with the recipe below) or use sour cream
2 tsp. Horseradish Dijon Mustard (or 1+ tsp. each horseradish + Dijon mustard)
Salt & pepper
2 Tbsp. finely diced red onion
Regular or smoked paprika

Boil and cool eggs as above. Carefully peel eggs, then cut in half length-wise. Scoop out yolks into a smaller bowl. Add remaining ingredients, except red onion and paprika. Blend using a fork to mash up the yolk. Spoon back into the egg whites. Sprinkle red onion and paprika on top.

Mayonnaise

1 egg + 1 egg yolk
Juice of 1/2 lemon
1/4 tsp. white pepper
1/2 tsp. cream of tartar

1/2 tsp. dry yellow mustard
Pinch of salt
1/2 tsp. sweetener, or pinch of stevia, optional
3/4-1 cup of single-sourced, mellow or floral flavored olive oil, or avocado oil

Place ingredients in a blender or food processor. Slowly pour in oil while continuing to blend until it coagulates and becomes thick and creamy. Add more oil if needed.

Also good for making chicken, turkey, or tuna salad, and/or coleslaw.

Eggnog

1.5-2 cups milk of choice
2-3 eggs
1-2 tsp. honey
1 Tbsp. bulk gelatin or collagen, or any other optional ingredients, below

Blend for 15 seconds in a blender.

Optional Ingredients:

- Instead of honey, add 1 packet Pruvit Keto Sweet Kreme ~ my favorite addition to the Eggnog
- Add 1 peach, or 1 cup of cantaloupe
- Add 1 tsp. real vanilla
- Add 1 tsp. cinnamon

- Add 1 tsp. cocoa powder
- Add a few squirts of Pruvit 1:4:3 oil, or 1/2-1 tsp. each coconut oil & MCT oil ~ the right ratio of both MCT & coconut oil allows the oil to remain liquid, hence the 1:4:3 formulation, with 4 parts MCT to 3 parts coconut oils, and 1 part phosphatidylserine (PS) which is a natural brain booster

Beef, Fish, Poultry & Pork

Several recipes can be used interchangeably with a variety of meats, which are included in parenthesis after the recipe name. Our **MEATS & SWEETS** approach is geared to being as *simple as possible.* Experiment, and modify as you see fit.

Meatballs with Asparagus Simmered in Tomato ~

During a recent visit with my mother, I made her a supply of the meatballs to freeze before leaving. She had picked up asparagus from her local farmers market, so this dish was the result.

Meatballs:

2 lbs. 85% lean ground beef, or a blend of grass-fed ground beef & pork
2 eggs (1 egg per pound of meat if using more meat)
1/2 sweet or yellow onion, diced
2 small cloves garlic, crushed
1/2 bunch (2 big handfuls) fresh parsley, chopped
2-3 Tbsp. raisins
Salt & pepper
2 tsp. oregano
1/2 tsp. ground fennel
1 tsp. sweetener of choice, or 1/4 tsp. cinnamon

Sauce:

2 Tbsp. XVOO or other cooking fat

1 bunch asparagus, ends trimmed and stalks cut into 2 -3 inch pieces
1 14.5 oz. can crushed Roma tomato (or your favorite)
2+ tsp. oregano
1 tsp. coconut or organic sugar, molasses, or honey, or tiny pinch of stevia
Big spoonful of fresh ricotta cheese, or parmesan cheese

Make the Meatballs:

Mash together meatball ingredients using your hands until well combined. Roll into balls. These can be fried, baked, or layered on wax or parchment paper, and frozen until ready to use.

If baking, place parchment paper on baking tray, and bake at ~ 375° until done, roughly 30 minutes.

Meatballs Simmered in Tomato Sauce:

Heat a large, deep pan. Add oil. When just hot, add raw meatballs. After a couple minutes, turn to continue to brown each side.

Add asparagus, and let cook for a few minutes before adding tomato. Cover, turn to medium to medium-low, and let simmer for 10-15 minutes. Garnish with a spoonful of ricotta or parmesan cheese.

Variations:

- Sub sliced mushrooms and sweet onion for asparagus, and cook as above.
- Simmer in beef bone broth with either half a small can of tomato paste, or a few fresh chopped Roma tomatoes, or skip tomatoes if not tolerated.
- Sub cabbage cut across like fettuccini for the asparagus.
- Make zucchini noodles using a mandolin or spiralizer to create long thin noodle shapes, then soften by letting noodles soak in heated water a few minutes. Top with meatballs, tomato sauce, and grated parmesan cheese.
- Skip the veg, enjoy the meatballs.

Meatloaf

You will need 1-2 baking dishes, depending on how much meat you use. I use either 2 8x8 baking dishes, or 1 plus 1 loaf pan for 3-4 pounds of meat.

2+ lbs. 85% lean ground beef (or your favorite ground meat)
1/2 large sweet onion, diced
1-2 small cloves garlic - remove inner green stems, then mince or crush with a garlic press
2 eggs
2+ tsp. salt
1 Tbsp. dried oregano

1 14.5 oz. can (or half a larger can) crushed tomatoes, divided
1 tsp.+ honey, molasses, coconut sugar, organic sugar, or sweetener of choice OR 1/8-1/4 tsp. cinnamon

Pre-heat oven to about 400°.

Using your hands, mash all ingredients together in a large mixing bowl until just combined, using about 1/3 of the can of tomatoes.

Place mixture into the baking dish or loaf pans. Place in oven and roast at the high temperature for just 5-10 minutes, then turn the heat down to 300° and bake for about one hour.

Meanwhile, pour the remaining crushed tomatoes into a small bowl. Add a pinch of salt, and sweetener. Stir, taste, and adjust flavor if needed. You just want to balance the acid flavor of the tomato with a little sweet, salty flavor. Add more oregano if desired.

When meatloaf is nearly cooked through, it will be nicely browned, with plenty of fat around the edges, and have a fairly firm texture.

Stab through several places on the top of the loaf with a small, thin knife to let some of the sauce sink in. Cover the tops of the loaves with the sauce.

Return to the oven for another 10 minutes. Remove, let cool, then cut and serve.

Meatloaf Variations:

- Add one peeled and grated zucchini to meatloaf mixture
- Add 1/4 cup (+/-) raisins, currants, or dried cranberries
- Sub 1/2+ bunch fresh, finely chopped parsley for the oregano, or use both
- Spice it up with a little cayenne, or white ground pepper
- Add any other vegetables you enjoy and well tolerate, such as shredded carrots (to sweeten) or chopped mushrooms

Sauce Variations:

- Sub garam masala for the cinnamon
- Sub ketchup or tomato paste for the crushed tomatoes; add fresh grated and squeezed ginger, (or 1/4+ tsp. dried, ground ginger), 1 tsp. dried yellow mustard, 2 tsp. brown sugar or other sweetener, and a splash of Coconut Aminos, or equivalent, instead of salt

Grain-Free Stuffed Peppers

4-6 even sized bell peppers, any color
2-3 lbs. 85% lean ground beef

2 eggs
1 sweet or yellow onion, diced or minced
3-4 garlic cloves, minced or crushed
1 tsp. each fennel seeds & fenugreek seeds, ground
1 tsp. each salt & cracked black pepper
1 Tbsp. each dried parsley and oregano
1 14.5-16 oz. can Italian tomato sauce, divided
2 tsp. sugar, or sweetener of choice

Preheat oven to 375° Have a baking dish, or Dutch oven pot ready.

Cut out a circle at the top of each pepper and remove the stem. Scoop out the seeds and pulp. Place peppers in a steamer basket and steam on medium heat for about 10 minutes until softer, but still a little firm. Remove from heat.

Place fennel and fenugreek seeds in a designated grinder to grind. (Omit if you don't have one or the other.)

Place ground beef in a large mixing bowl. Add remaining ingredients including 1/3 of the can of tomato sauce, and 1/2-1 full teaspoon of sugar. Work the mixture with your hands until everything is well combined.

When peppers are cool enough to handle, spoon in meat mixture. Fill to top, gently pressing it in without breaking the pepper. Fit peppers upright snuggly into your baking dish or pot. Stir 1/2-1 tsp. sugar into remaining tomato sauce, then pour over peppers. Sprinkle more oregano on top.

If using a baking dish, cover peppers with foil. If using a Dutch oven, cover with lid, then place in oven. Bake for about one hour. Let cool a bit, serve and enjoy!

Grilled Sirloin (or other Steaks) with Sautéed Onions & Mushrooms

Steaks of choice
Balsamic vinegar & XVOO
Salt & pepper

Pre-marinate steaks by placing on a plate, or in a baking dish. Drizzle balsamic vinegar and XVOO on top, and season with salt and pepper. Let sit 1 hour to overnight in the fridge. When ready to prepare, let sit out at room temperature for 10+ minutes before grilling. Grill to desired doneness.

Sautéed Onions & Mushrooms

1 Tbsp. each XVOO + butter for cooking
1 lg. sweet or yellow onion, sliced
1 8 oz. pack of mushrooms, any variety, chopped or sliced
Italian seasoning or oregano
2 tsp. balsamic vinegar

Heat a large sauté pan, and add XVOO & butter. When hot, add onions. Season with salt and pepper. After a few minutes, add mushrooms. Season with more salt and pepper, and Italian seasoning. Let cook on medium heat for 20+ minutes, until onions are well cooked. Add balsamic vinegar, stir through, and let cook another few minutes. Serve on steaks.

Quick Beef 'Stroganoff' ~ *I'm calling this Stroganoff, but it's not quite. If desired, add sour cream instead of half and half. Who needs the noodles? It's just a great way to use already prepared roast beef.*

Prepare Sautéed Onions & Mushrooms as above, using generous amounts of a variety of mushrooms. I recently made this with baby bellas, shiitakes, and chanterelle mushrooms.

Once cooked through, after adding vinegar, add diced already cooked/leftover roast beef, and some half and half ~ about 1/4 cup or a bit more. Stir, and let heat through on medium-low heat. Serve in a shallow bowl and enjoy.

Lime Marinated Pork Chops (Or Chicken or Fish)

2-4 servings of center cut boneless pork chops (or try with mild or meaty white fish, Keta or wild salmon, chicken breast or thighs, or turkey thighs)
Juice of 2+ limes
2-3 Tbsp. XVOO
Salt & white or black pepper
Garlic powder, optional
2 tsp. each butter + XVOO for cooking

Prepare in advance:

Place meat in a shallow baking dish. Add remaining ingredients, except for cooking fat. Toss meat to evenly coat. Refrigerate one hour to overnight.

When ready to prepare, pat meat dry. Warm a pan on medium, or a little higher heat. Add cooking fat. Once heated, add meat and cook a few minutes.

Once the pork chops begin to brown, turn over. Turn heat down a bit if needed, and continue to cook until cooked through. If using fish, turn once the fish becomes more opaque. Fish will cook faster, so do pay attention. Poultry will need to cook longer.

Try not to over cook to avoid drying out meat. Pork will have a glistening white to slightly pinkish color, and an internal temperature of about 135-140°; chicken should be white, with clear juices and an internal temperature of 150-160°; and fish should easily flake with a fork.

Serve with stewed apples and raisins, apple sauce, or sautéed vegetables.

Pesto Chicken (Or Pork or Meatier White Fish)

2-4 boneless, skinless chicken breasts, lean pork chops, or firm white fish, such as wild caught mahi mahi, halibut, or cod
Juice of 1 lemon or 2 limes
1 Tbsp. XVOO
Sea salt and pepper
2 tsp. each butter & XVOO for cooking
1/2 cup or more Parsley Pesto or Basil Pesto

If using thicker chicken breasts, cut in half width-wise. It may be easier to cut when slightly frozen. If able, cover chicken with Saran wrap, then pound on a cutting board to create more even-sized pieces.

Place chicken, pork, or fish in a shallow baking dish, and add lemon or lime juice, XVOO, salt and pepper. Let marinate for 1 hour.

When ready to cook, warm a pan on medium to medium-high heat. Add oil and butter. Once the fat has heated, add chicken or pork. Turn over once it begins to brown. If using fish, it will start to look more opaque.

Continue to cook until nearly cooked through ~ about 7 more minutes for chicken or pork, less for fish. Add pesto sauce. Turn to medium-low, cover, and simmer for 3-5 minutes.

Alternatively, keep meat in the baking pan, cover with pesto sauce, and bake at 325-350° for anywhere between 10 minutes for fish, to 20 minutes for chicken. For moister meat, cover loosely with foil before baking.

Parsley Pesto

1/2+ bunch of parsley, big stems removed
Juice of 1 lemon
1/4+ cup grated parmesan cheese (or sub 2 Tbsp. nutritional yeast)
1 clove garlic
Pinch each of sea salt & pepper
Pinch of cayenne pepper, or dash of hot sauce, optional
1/4 cup+ XVOO, or avocado, hazelnut, macadamia, or pecan oil

Place all ingredients except for the oil in a food processor. Pulse a few times, then continue to blend while slowly pouring in the oil. Taste, and adjust flavor as needed.

Basil Pesto

Presoak 2 sun-dried tomatoes in water

4 cups basil, loosely packed
Juice of 1 lemon
1-2 small cloves garlic
1/4+ cup parmesan cheese (or sub 2 Tbsp. nutritional yeast)
2 rehydrated sun-dried tomatoes plus 2 tsp. soaking liquid
Salt & pepper
Pinch of red pepper flakes, or dash of hot sauce, optional
1 tsp. sweetener of choice
1/4 cup+ XVOO, or hazelnut or pecan oil

Place ingredients except oil in a food processor. Pulse a few times, then continue to blend while slowly adding oil. Blend until well combined, adding more oil as needed. Taste, and adjust seasoning as needed.

Coconut-Herb Pan-Fried Chicken (Or Salmon)

When pan-frying chicken breast, it will cook more evenly if the chicken breasts are about 1/2 inch thick in width. An easy way to cut plump chicken breasts in half width-wise is to freeze for up to one hour before cutting. Otherwise, cover with saran wrap, place on a wooden cutting board, and beat the breast down with a mallet.

2-4 skinless, boneless chicken breasts, chicken tenders, or salmon filets
1 egg
1/2 cup coconut flour
2 Tbsp. Herbs De Provence (French herb blend with a little lavender) or a blend of dried thyme, basil, & oregano
Couple pinches of cayenne pepper
Sea salt and cracked pepper
1 Tbsp. each butter & coconut oil for cooking

Cut chicken breasts in half width-wise, as outlined above. Whisk egg in a small, shallow bowl. Use a fork to mix coconut flour, herbs, and seasonings together on a separate plate or shallow bowl.

Heat a cast iron, or stainless steel pan, or flat-top griddle. Add coconut oil and butter. Dip chicken in egg, then herb mixture, turning to fully coat. Place into pan when the cooking fat is hot enough for the meat to sizzle.

Cook until nicely browned, flip, then cook until nicely browned on the other side, and cooked through, roughly 10-12 minutes on medium heat, quicker for salmon.

Try not to over cook so the meat stays moist, and doesn't dry out. It should feel fairly firm, but with a little give when pressing with a finger. Salmon should easily flake.

Curry Chicken (Or Cod or other Meaty White Fish)

1-2 lbs. chicken tenders or cod filets, or 2-4 chicken breasts or thighs
Salt & white or black pepper
1 Tbsp. sweet curry spice powder, or turmeric + a little sweetener
1 Tbsp. each butter + coconut oil
Wedge of lemon

If using thicker chicken breasts, cut in half widthwise so they are thinner and more uniform in size. Cut into chicken tender sized pieces, or leave as is. If using thighs, leave whole.

Place chicken or cod on a big platter, and season with salt, pepper, and curry.

Heat a pan and add butter and oil. When hot, add chicken or cod. Turn once it begins to brown. Brown the other side, then simmer on lower heat until done.

To test for doneness, chicken tenders should be firm, with a slight give upon pressing. If using whole chicken thighs, cover after turning over, and let simmer until cooked through. If needed, remove one and cut in half to check for doneness. Cod will be opaque and easily flake once ready.

Ketchup Chicken

Ketchup is the perfect tangy, yet sweet acid marinade for chicken breast. It helps break down the muscle fibers, and tenderizes the meat.

1-2 lbs. chicken tenders, breast, or thighs
Several squirts of ketchup
1-2 Tbsp. XVOO
2 tsp. balsamic vinegar
1 tsp. coconut sugar or maple syrup
1/3 tsp. salt
1/3 tsp. white pepper
1/8 tsp. each of garam masala and cinnamon
Pinch of cayenne, or drizzle of hot sauce, optional
1 Tbsp. each butter or ghee + coconut oil or XVOO (for cooking)

Place the chicken in a baking dish. Add a few squirts of ketchup, plus remaining ingredients except the cooking fat. Massage in to evenly coat. Let sit for one hour to overnight in the fridge.

Heat a pan, and add cooking fat. When the chicken begins to look white around the edges, turn over, and continue to cook until firm with a little give when pressed, and still tender but cooked through.

Alternatively, try grilling chicken, and add the Barbecue Sauce, below.

Quick Homemade Barbecue Sauce

About 1/2 cup ketchup or tomato paste
1/4 tsp. salt, or 1-2 tsp. Coconut Aminos
3/4 tsp. dry yellow mustard
2+ tsp. brown sugar, maple syrup, or honey
Pinch of dried ginger, optional
Few drops of liquid smoke, optional
Few drops liquid hot sauce, optional

Stir ingredients and taste test. Adjust if needed with more sweetness, salty flavor, or spice.

Baste onto grilled chicken the last 5-10 minutes of cooking.

Pineapple Chicken Stir-Fry

1-2 lbs. chicken breast, cut into bite-sized chunks

Marinade:
Juice of 1 lemon, 2 limes, 1/2 white grapefruit, OR 2 Tbsp. apple cider vinegar
2 Tbsp. XVOO
Salt & white or black pepper
2 tsp. garlic herb seasoning
1 tsp. turmeric, optional

1 Tbsp. each butter + coconut oil
1-2 stalks celery, sliced on the bias
2 scallions, sliced on an angle (on the bias)

1 zucchini, cut in half moons or long thin shapes
2-3 rings pineapple from a can + 1 Tbsp. juice
1 tsp. honey, coconut sugar, or brown sugar

Pre-marinate chicken by placing chicken pieces in a baking dish or large ziplock bag, along with marinade ingredients. Toss chicken if in a baking dish, or close bag and massage to fully coat. Let sit one hour to overnight in the fridge.

Heat a wok on medium-high heat. Add oil. Add celery, and stir with a wooden spatula. After a minute or two, add chicken. Continue to stir fry on higher heat.

After a couple minutes, add the rest of the vegetables. Keep stirring, until chicken is tender, but firm and nearly cooked through.

Tear pineapple rings up into smaller pieces as you add them to the stir fry, along with pineapple juice, and sweetener. Let cook another few minutes, until chicken is cooked through, but still tender.

Ceviche

1 lb. raw wild caught cod or other mild white fish, or salmon
2 limes
2-3 Tbsp. XVOO
Salt & pepper

1 scallion, finely diced (or 1/4 red onion)
Several grape or other small tomatoes, halved or quartered
1 tsp. sugar, optional
Pinch of cayenne, optional
2-3 inch piece of dulse, cut into small pieces, or dulse flakes, garnish

Cut fish up into 1 inch pieces, and place in a bowl. Add remaining ingredients. Let sit one hour or longer in the refrigerator. The citrus 'cooks' the fish, and turns it more opaque in color. Garnish with dulse flakes.

Raw Liver with Cocktail Sauce

1-2 oz. raw, or frozen calves liver per serving
1+ tsp. each ketchup and horseradish

Cut liver into smaller pieces, and toss with ketchup and horseradish.

Seared Liver

4 oz. calves liver, cut into 2 inch pieces, or use chicken livers
Garlic salt & pepper
Butter for cooking

Heat skillet on medium-high. Add butter. Season liver, then add to pan. Once browned, turn. Cook briefly until browned on both sides, and slightly tender when pressed. When cooked right, liver should still be tender tasting, rather than dry and mealy. It's much better if not over cooked!

Chicken livers will have a mousse-like texture, however, if you prefer them to be firmer, cook longer as desired.

Slow Roasting Method

Basic Slow Roast Beef Recipe

Beef roast of choice
~1/3 cup Balsamic vinegar
2 Tbsp. olive oil (XVOO)
1-2 cloves garlic, crushed
Salt & pepper
Fresh ground rosemary + cumin seeds
1/2 cup bone broth or water

Pre-heat oven to 425°
Place roast in roasting pan. Combine remaining ingredients, except for bone broth/water, in a small bowl. Use a pastry brush to brush all over the roast. Add broth or water to the pan.

Roast at 425° for 15-20 minutes, then reduce heat to 250-275° and roast for 4+ hours. Check on it half way through to baste if able, but not necessary. If dry, add a bit more broth or water. Remove from heat, and let cool before slicing.

Notes:

- In lieu of using XVOO, you can also use a butter knife to spread some beef tallow on top, or leave a couple teaspoons worth in the roasting pan. The fat on top of the roast will help it brown quickly, so do be careful.

- To keep it uber simple, simply cover top of vinegar bottle with one finger, and shake drops all over roast. Do the same with the olive oil. Season generously, and roast as above.
- Pay attention to the aroma, or set a timer to not over roast it at the higher temperature!
- The beef can roast for up to 4-6 hours. Just keep heat low, but not too low your oven will turn itself off if you will be away from home while it roasts. Or use a slow cooker, and follow roasting instructions.
- If you need it quicker than 6 hours, roast at 300°.

Super Flavorful Pulled Beef

1 2-4 lb. leaner beef roast (rump, bottom or top round)
1 sweet or yellow onion, cut into wedges or rings
Garlic salt or powder, salt & pepper
3/4-1 cup Concord grape juice
1/4 cup balsamic vinegar
About 2 Tbsp. beef tallow or other cooking fat

Pre-heat oven to 400°

Heat an oven-proof pot or Dutch oven on medium-high heat. Add cooking fat. Season meat well, then place in pot, along with onion. When meat just begins to brown, turn, and cook until seared, or slightly brown on all sides. Add juice and vinegar.

Cover, and place in oven. Roast for about 15 minutes, then reduce heat to 250° and roast for another 4+ hours.

Remove from oven and let cool for several minutes. Use a fork to tear meat apart, like a pulled beef. It should be fork tender, and smell amazing!

Slow Roast Turkey Breast

Turkey breast is a lean meat that benefits from a dry brine. (A wet brine would involve leaving it in a bucket of salt water.)

Place the turkey breast in your roasting pan. Squeeze fresh orange or lemon all over, which helps tenderize the meat. Generously season with salt **all over**, and any poultry seasonings you like, such as dried sage or thyme. Let it sit *uncovered* in the fridge over night. It can sit there a couple days if needed.

Pre-heat oven to 400-425°. When it comes time to roasting a leaner meat like turkey breast, I will add pats of butter all over the breast, especially under the skin.

Roast turkey uncovered for 15-20 minutes, or roughly five minutes per pound. Once it starts to get a little browned on top, turn the heat down to about 275-300°, and roast for 2-3 hours for a smaller breast, longer if bigger. A thermometer inserted at the thickest area should measure 145-150° or a bit more, and the juices should run clear.

Add a loose foil tent over the breast if it starts to get too brown, later in the roasting process.

Keeping it uncovered will net crispier skin. If you prefer an even moister finish, loosely cover throughout the roasting process. It will be juicier, but the skin will not be crisp.

Alternatively, roast it covered on the low heat the entire time, then remove the foil cover, and roast on higher heat for the last 30 minutes to help brown and crisp up the skin. A reversed slow roast.

Slow Roast Chicken or Turkey with Apple

1 4-7 lb. whole chicken or turkey breast
1 sweet or yellow onion, cut into 1/4 inch wedges
1 green or other apple, peeled and sliced into wedges
1+ celery stalk, cut into 3-4 inch pieces
1 lemon or orange
Several pats of butter
1/4 cup apple juice, water, or bone broth
Salt, pepper, dried thyme, ground sage

Pre-heat oven to 400-425°

Place apple + vegetables in the bottom of a roasting pan or large baking dish, and fit chicken or turkey on top.

Cut lemon or orange into quarters. Squeeze juice all around chicken or turkey. Put what remains into the cavity, or toss. Season generously with dried herbs, salt and pepper.

If able, peel back some of the skin and wedge butter pats inside the skin, or just on top of, around, and inside breast cavity.

Roast uncovered at high temperature for 15-20 minutes, as above, then turn heat down to about 300°, and carefully add apple juice, water or bone broth. Continue to roast at lower heat for 2-3 hours, basting every hour. Tent foil over the top towards the last hour if getting too brown.

Check temperature at the leg, or thickest area of the chicken or turkey. If roasting a whole bird, the leg should easily twist off, and juices should come out clear. The internal temperature should be 150 - 165°. Remove from oven, and let cool before cutting.

Lamb Shanks (or sub Beef Shank or Oxtail)

Crock pot or large Le Creuset Dutch Oven Pot (or similar)

Cooking fat (~ 1 Tbsp. beef tallow, or XVOO +/- butter)
2+ lamb shanks, or 2 lbs. beef shank or ox tail
Salt or garlic salt & pepper
3/4 tsp. paprika
1/3 tsp. garam masala **or** 1/4 tsp. cinnamon
1/4 tsp. dried rosemary (or more if not ground)
1/2+ sweet or yellow onion, cut in chunks
1-2 carrots, chopped
1 celery stalk, sliced
1-2 cloves garlic cut lengthwise into quarters
1 small butternut squash, peeled, seeded and cut into cubes (or 1-2 cups frozen and thawed) or 1 small sweet potato, peeled and chopped
6 prunes
1 cup beef bone broth or consommé
1 14.5 oz. can crushed or petite Roma or Italian tomatoes

If using a Crockpot, turn to high to begin to warm. If using a dutch oven, turn oven to 400°.

Season shanks (or ox tail if using) with salt and/or garlic salt and pepper. Heat a big pan, or the dutch oven, and add cooking fat. Brown shanks or ox tail, turning as it begins to brown to quickly sear each side. Add paprika, garam masala or cinnamon, and rosemary, and stir to coat the meat.

If using a Crockpot, add onion, carrot, and celery. Add lamb shanks or meat, followed by remaining ingredients. Cook on high about one hour, then reduce to low setting. Let cook 5-6 hours. (Adjust settings as needed.)

If using the dutch oven, add remaining ingredients, nestling the meat into the vegetables. Place in oven. Turn heat down to ~275° and let roast 5-6 hours. It can roast all day.

Notes:

Adjust this recipe as you desire. The prunes and squash or sweet potato provide a nice sweet balance to the tomato broth and the meat. Use what you prefer, eliminating any as you see fit. If tomatoes are off the menu, just increase the beef broth. If using store bought beef broth, check sodium content, reducing salt added to the meat as needed. Sub a little molasses, sweetener, or raisins for the prunes.

Slow Roast Chicken (or Beef or Pork Roast) with Tomato & Onion

Cooking fat ~ beef tallow, ghee, or fat of choice
1 sweet onion, coarse chopped
2-4 bone-in chicken breasts (or thighs), or 1 2-3 lb. beef or pork roast
1+ cup canned crushed Roma tomatoes
Salt and pepper
Italian seasoning blend
1/2+ cup bone broth, or soup stock
Handful of pitted and chopped black olives, optional

Preheat oven to 450°

Heat a dutch oven or oven-proof pot, and add cooking fat. When heated, add onion, and sauté until onion begins to soften.

Place chicken or roast on top of onions, and season with salt and pepper. Cook a few minutes, then turn to briefly cook each side.

Add tomatoes and broth. Generously season with Italian seasoning. Add olives if using.

Cover pot, and place in oven. After about 10 minutes, turn heat to about 250°, and let it slow roast 3-4 hours, until the chicken (or beef or pork roast) are tender enough to pull apart with a fork. When cool enough to handle, use a fork to pull apart meat if able, otherwise, cut/slice as desired and serve in a shallow bowl with tomato and onion sauce on top.

Variations:

- Add 2 cups sauerkraut when adding tomatoes
- Use whole or ground rosemary and fennel seeds in addition to or in lieu of Italian seasoning
- For sweetness, sub 5-6 prunes for the olives

Honey Baked Drumsticks

6 chicken or 2+ turkey drumsticks
A few thin shavings of butter
3 Tbsp. coconut oil, XVOO, or pecan oil
1/2-1 Tbsp. rice vinegar, or juice of 1/2 an orange
1-2 Tbsp. honey
1/2+ tsp. chili garlic sauce
1/3 tsp. sea salt

Preheat oven to 400°.

Place chicken drumsticks in an 8x8 glass or ceramic baking dish. Spread shavings of butter around, adding a small piece to the top of each drumstick. Place chicken in the oven, and roast for 30 minutes.

Meanwhile, combine remaining ingredients in a small bowl. Do a quick taste test to see if it needs a tad more sweet, sour, or salty flavor.

Turn drumsticks over, then pour honey sauce on top. Return to oven, and reduce temperature to 375°.

Bake for another 30 minutes, until the meat easily tears off the bone. Remove from oven, and use a big spoon to ladle some of the sauce on the chicken drumsticks when serving.

Citrus Roasted Chicken (or Turkey) Thighs

4 chicken or 2 turkey thighs
2 lemons
3 Tbsp. olive oil
Salt, and cracked black pepper
1-2 Tiny pinches of cayenne pepper
Generous amount of dried Greek oregano, thyme, and parsley

Preheat oven to 400°.

Place chicken or turkey thighs in 8x8 glass baking dish, skin side up. In a small bowl, combine juice of lemon or lime, olive oil, and seasonings. Baste over the chicken or turkey using a pastry brush. Add more dried herbs to the thighs so there is good coverage.

Place thighs in oven, and roast for 30 minutes, then reduce heat to 375° and roast for another 35-40 minutes for chicken, or one hour for turkey.

Insert a meat thermometer to test for doneness. The internal temperature should be near 160°. You can also test by cutting into one of the thighs near the fattest part. Any juices released should be clear, and the meat should be cooked through. If it is shiny or glossy, or very pink towards the bone, cook another 10 or so minutes.

Variations:

- Sub melted butter, ghee, or coconut oil for the olive oil
- If using coconut oil instead of the olive oil, try with lime juice instead of lemon
- Sub apple cider vinegar, or apple juice for the citrus, and add a little sweet yellow curry powder or turmeric, along with the dried herbs
- Crank up the heat by adding a little hot sauce
- Pre-marinate by placing chicken or turkey thighs into a big ziplock bag. Add lemon, oil, seasonings and herbs, plus optional hot sauce. Close bag, then massage to fully coat the chicken thighs. Marinate one hour to overnight, then place in an oven and roast as above.

Bone Broth & Soups

Super Gelatinous Pressure-Cooked Bone Broth

Save bones and carcasses from any meals with bones including steaks, bone-in chicken or turkey ~ whole or parts ~ including legs, thighs, necks, tails and breasts in the freezer until ready to use. Purchase chicken feet, or toes or tails of animals, such as ox tail for super gelatinous-rich bone broth.

When ready to make bone broth, fill up a pressure cooker (or Insta-Pot) 2/3 full of bones. If using chicken feet, oxtail, or toes, just a couple along with other bones should be adequate. If using whole chicken, place the entire chicken into the pot, still adding 1-2 chicken feet if available.

Cover bones with pure water, leaving two inches, or whatever may be marked as the full line in your cooker. Add juice of half a lemon, or 2 tablespoons of apple cider vinegar (pulls minerals out of the bones, into the broth) plus a 4 to 6 inch piece of seaweed, such as alaria, kombu, or kelp, to add iodine, and other minerals. Close lid tightly, and bring up to pressure on medium-high heat. Once up to pressure, reduce heat to about a medium to medium-low, and let simmer for one or more hours. Insta pots may take less cooking time.

Turn off heat and let fully come down from pressure before opening the lid. When cool enough, strain out bones, then pour broth into jars. Let cool uncovered several minutes before refrigerating. Once chilled, it should create a nice thick layer of fat at the top, which preserves the broth.

If pot simmering (instead of pressure cooking) keep lid slightly ajar. Cook at a medium heat for the first two hours, then turn low and let it simmer, 3-4 more hours, longer if desired. Pay attention to water level and add more if needed.

Notes: I like to add a handful each of dried cranberries and dried rose hips to beef bones as it adds a nice flavor, plus it boosts the vitamin C. Alternatively add up to an entire bunch of fresh parsley to the broth before closing the lid.

Fish heads are also make an excellent broth, especially good for making chowders or try the Fish Soup, below.

Fish Soup

3 cups bone broth, ideally made with fish head and bones
1 Tbsp. each XVOO + butter
1 sweet onion, chopped, or cut in half moon shapes
2 stalks celery, diced, or cut in thin slices on an angle
1 carrot, chopped

Several shiitake, chanterelle, or white button mushrooms, sliced, optional
1 tsp. turmeric
1 tsp. dill or marjoram
Salt and pepper
1 can drained smoked oysters, or other fish of choice, cut into 1 inch chunks
1 cup whole milk
2+ oz. muenster cheese, cut into chunks
2 inch piece of dulse seaweed, cut into small strips

Place bone broth into a pot, and bring to a gentle simmer while preparing vegetables.

Heat a separate deep pan, and add XVOO + butter. Once heated, add onion, cook for a minute, then add celery, carrot, and seasonings. Stir and cook several minutes, until vegetables soften.

Add oysters or fish, and stir to fully integrate. Turn down heat a little and add broth, then milk. Once the milk heats, you can either add cheese into the pot, or ladle into serving bowls, and add cheese to each bowl. Garnish each bowl with dulse strips.

Alternatively, heat dulse first in a toaster oven, or frying pan to crisp it up. Use a medium to low heat, and pay attention, as it only requires a couple minutes of heat before it will burn. Crumble or cut into each bowl. Tastes a bit like bacon when added to the fish soup.

Creamy Mushroom Soup *Several folks in the Ray Peat forums boil mushrooms for 1+ hour, in order to extract all the nutrients. You can either do that, or simply sauté mushrooms in fat first.*

1+ lbs. of mushrooms ~ use white button, baby bellas, shiitakes, chanterelles, morels, or your favorites
Bone broth or water
Salt and pepper
2 tsp. thyme, Greek oregano, or Italian seasoning
1 tsp. rosemary
Half and half
Optional: hot sauce, sour cream, cubed roast beef

Place whole mushrooms in a pot, and add enough bone broth or water to just cover. Simmer on medium for one hour. Check periodically to ensure there is enough liquid to avoid scorching.

After one hour, it should be mostly mushrooms, with a tiny bit of broth remaining. Season with salt and pepper, and remaining seasoning.

Blend all at once or in batches with some half and half, to desired creaminess. I did not add a precise amount as it will depend on how much you've made, and how much half and half you prefer. I would say start with about 1/4 cup at a time, adding more as desired to taste. Do a quick taste test, and adjust seasoning if needed.

Pour back into pot to warm gently a few minutes. Serve as is, or with a splash of hot sauce, dollop of sour cream, and/or add cubed leftover roast beef.

Alternatively, sauté mushrooms in butter until soft, then season and purée with half and half as above.

Carrot Apple Ginger Soup

1 Tbsp. coconut oil, or 1/2 Tbsp. each coconut oil & butter or ghee
1 lb. or 6 carrots, peeled and chopped
1/4 inch piece of ginger, minced or 1 inch piece of ginger, peeled & grated
1/8 tsp. each coriander & allspice
Sea salt & cracked pepper
1-1&1/2 tart (granny smith or honeycrisp) apples, peeled & chopped
1 cup apple juice or cider
About 1/2 cup canned coconut milk, & 1/4-1/3 cup half and half, or use just one or the other, but I like the blend of both for more balanced flavor

Add oil &/or butter or ghee to a heavy-bottomed pot. When heated, add carrots. Squeeze ginger if grated to add the juice, or if minced, add to pot, followed by the coriander, allspice, and a couple pinches each of salt and pepper. Stir to combine. After a couple minutes, add apple, then juice or cider. Simmer on medium, loosely covered, until carrots are soft.

Here you have a choice. Add coconut milk and half and half, stir and heat through. Turn off the heat. Carefully ladle into blender in batches if needed, blending a good minute until creamy and smooth. I often just add soup with enough of the coconut milk or half and half in each batch directly to the blender, combining it all at the end.

I like the flavor of the combination of half and half and coconut milk, but if you love coconut milk, skip the half and half, or if you don't like coconut milk, use half and half, and/or milk.

You could also try the above soup subbing kabocha or butternut squash for the carrots. Peel, and cut into chunks, cooking as above until soft. Or bake first, and separately simmer the apples and spices in the juice, blending everything together at the end.

More Quick Soups

Once you have bone broth made, quick soups are a breeze. Here are a couple ideas:

- Heat broth, and add leftover cut up chicken, turkey, or roast pork or beef, diced tomato, and thin sliced scallions.
- Add sautéed thick sliced sweet onion and mushrooms to heated broth. Season with salt, garlic, and oregano, and add leftover diced meat, or canned and drained smoked oysters, as desired.
- Heat broth, and add 1-2 eggs right into the soup. Vigorously stir eggs in broth with a fork. Alternatively, scramble eggs in a bowl first. Another option is to fry the eggs separately, then add on top of soup. Top with grated or shaved parmesan cheese. Also good with a squeeze of lemon.
- If craving something starchy, use broth for cooking potatoes. Make into a quick soup by adding garlic, and sliced celery, and/or roast green chilis. Or cook potatoes, and mash them as desired with milk, salt, white pepper, and optional chives.

5 - SWEETS
Fruit Salads, Jello Recipes & Other Treats

Fruit is the quintessentially ideal 'fast food.' I'm not a baker as I prefer to get my sweet fixe primarily with fresh or dried fruit, honey, or a little real maple syrup. Warmed milk sweetened with maple syrup or honey is a great treat before bed, and may aid sleep. Life is meant to be sweet, and some of our sweetest memories are gatherings shared with family and friends.

Fruit Salads

Purple Power

1+ cup plain yogurt
2 tsp. raw/local honey
1+ cup purple grapes
3+ oz. blackberries
1+ Tbsp. finely shredded coconut, optional
2 squirts Pruvit 1:4:3 oil, or 1/2 tsp. each coconut & MCT oil, optional

Stir honey into yogurt in a serving bowl. Add fruit, and top with coconut if using, or place fruit in a bowl, top with yogurt and coconut, then drizzle honey on top.

Gingered Fruit

Fruit of choice, but especially good with grapes, apricots, pineapple, melon, papaya, and mango
2 inch piece of ginger
Few leaves of basil or mint, thinly sliced
Squeeze lemon, lime, or orange
2 tsp. honey, more or less to taste
Tiny pinch of salt, optional

Place fruit in a bowl. Peel, grate, and squeeze ginger over the fruit to get ginger juice. Add fresh juice, herbs (basil or mint), and honey, and toss to combine. Enjoy fruit as is, with yogurt, or with meat. Good after it sits.

Tropical Fruit Salad

Ripe papaya when available, cut into chunks
Mango, cut into chunks
1+ cup plain yogurt
2 tsp. honey
1+ Tbsp. unsweetened shredded coconut
2 squirts Pruvit 1:4:3 oil, or 1 tsp. each coconut and MCT oil

Combine all ingredients in a bowl, similar to Purple Power recipe above.

Grape + Apricot

1+ cup green grapes
1-2 fresh apricots, cut into chunks
1+ cup plain yogurt
2 tsp. honey or real maple syrup
Optional: Fresh fig if/when available; unsweetened finely shredded coconut; 2 squirts Pruvit 1:4:3 oil, or 1 tsp. each coconut & MCT oil

Combine ingredients in a bowl, and enjoy.

Cottage Cheese & Pineapple

1 cup cottage cheese (2% or 4%)
3 canned, unsweetened pineapple rings, cut in chunks
1 tsp. cinnamon
1 tsp. honey

Place cottage cheese in serving bowl. Top with remaining ingredients.

Variations:

- Sub raisins for the pineapple
- Sub raisins and 1/2 peeled and chopped apple
- Sub chopped peaches for the pineapple
- Sub rehydrated (soaked dried plums/prunes) for the pineapple, and add a little of the soaking juice (Especially good when adding a cinnamon stick to the soaking liquid. After days it gets thick, syrupy, and sweet!)

Waldorf Salad

1 each apple & pear, peeled and chopped
1-2 stalks celery, sliced
Juice of 1/2 a lemon
4+ soaked/rehydrated chopped dried plums (prunes) &/or raisins or dates, and a little of the soaking liquid
Tiny pinch of sea salt (optional)
1 tsp. cinnamon
1+ tsp. honey

Toss all ingredients in a bowl, and enjoy. About 4 servings. Will keep for day or two in the fridge.

Basic Stewed Apple Recipe

4 apples, peeled and chopped
Enough water (or apple cider) to just cover the bottom of a pot
Pinch of salt
About 1 tsp. cinnamon
Pinch of ground clove &/or cardamom
1/2+ cup fresh frozen or dried cranberries or raisins, or 4-5 prunes
2 tsp. honey or maple syrup, more or less to taste

Place ingredients in the pot, and bring to a gentle boil. Cover, reduce heat to medium-low, and simmer until apples are soft.

Variations:

- Add dried apricots in addition, or in lieu of any of the dried fruit
- Keep fruit whole or purée
- Enjoy stewed fruit topped with yogurt, or with meats

Cranberry Apricot Sauce

2 cups whole frozen or thawed cranberries
4-6 dried apricots
1/8 cup dried cranberries
1/8 cup raisins or currants
Water to cover
Pinch each of cinnamon & nutmeg, or clove
Honey or maple syrup to taste

Simmer ingredients in a pot on medium to medium-low heat, until the cranberries pop, and all the fruit softens. Strain into a food processor or blender, with as much cooking liquid as needed to blend into a thick sauce.

Cranberry Apple Sauce

2 cups fresh or frozen and thawed cranberries
4-5 medium apples, peeled and chopped
~2/3 cup raisins
1/4 tsp. sea salt
Water ~ up to 1/2 cup (or use apple juice or cider)

1 tbsp. arrowroot or kudzu dissolved in 2 tbsp. cool water

Layer all but the arrowroot in a large saucepan, and bring to a boil. Reduce heat to low, and simmer 30-35 minutes, without stirring. A heat deflector will help prevent scorching at the bottom.

Add arrowroot mixture to the pot, and simmer a few more minutes until mixture thickens. Using a potato masher or the back of a wooden spoon, mash the fruit mixture while stirring. It can remain somewhat lumpy. Blend in a food processor or blender if preferred. Let cool to set. Serve with turkey or have for breakfast with yogurt.

Try any of the following fruit combos. Follow the same instructions, subbing the seasonal fruit for the cranberries:

- **Peach Apple Sauce** ~ Sub 2-3 peaches for the cranberries
- **Pear, Apple, & Prune Sauce** ~ Use 2 each apple + pear, and 5 prunes instead of the raisins
- **Apple Cherry Sauce** ~ Sub 1-2 cups fresh pitted, or 1/2 cup dried cherries for the cranberries, and use 2-3 sweeter apples. Also good with grated and squeezed ginger juice, or cinnamon and a pinch of clove or nutmeg
- **Cranberry Orange** ~ Blend 2 cups whole cranberries in a food processor with 1 peeled

orange, 1/4 cup maple syrup, honey, or sugar, more or less to taste, and optional pinch cinnamon & nutmeg, or ginger juice. Enjoy as is, or gently simmer in a splash of water or juice before serving. Very refreshing!

Jello Recipes

Basic Jello Preparation

1 cup cold juice or water
3 Tbsp. bulk gelatin or 2-3 packets unflavored gelatin
2 cups juice, heated to near boiling
1+ tsp. honey, sugar or coconut sugar or 2 pinches of stevia
Fruit, optional

Add cold juice or water to a glass or ceramic bowl. Whisk in gelatin. This flowers the gelatin. (Using juice makes it sweeter, and more flavorful.)

Add heated juice and whisk well 1 minute to fully dissolve gelatin. Add sweetener if using, and let sit for 5 minutes. Add fruit if using, then refrigerate to set. Use a little less gelatin for less stiff jello.

Grape Jello

1 cup cold Concord grape juice, apple juice, or water
3 Tbsp. bulk gelatin
2 cups Concord grape juice, heated to near boiling
1+ packet Pruvit Purple Reign grape flavored exogenous ketones, optional
1+ tsp. honey or sugar, optional

Add cold juice or water to a glass or ceramic bowl. Whisk in gelatin, then ketone packet if using. Let sit while heating the remaining juice. When hot, but not boiling, add heated juice and whisk well, one minute. Taste test, and add sweetener if desired. Let sit 5 minutes, then refrigerate.

Variations for Juice-Based Jello Recipes:

- Sub cherry juice for the Concord grape juice
- Add the juice of a lime to add some tartness
- Try any other of your favorite juices, such as peach or apricot nectar, mango, or even various brewed herbal teas, such as our Rose Hips Tea, or others, however, fresh or frozen pineapple juice is not recommended

NOTE:

The Pruvit Purple Reign Grape Flavored is a perfect match with the Concord Grape Juice, however, it is not always available. You can omit the Pruvit ketones if you don't have them, or try with a different flavor, such as any of the recipes below using Maui Punch, Splash, or Heart Tart which are all excellent. See Resource section for more information. Ketones come either 'charged' which is equivalent of 1 cup of coffee, or caffeine-free.

Strawberry Apple ~ Fruit + Juice Jello ~ *I like using frozen and thawed strawberries for this recipe. I let the strawberries thaw in a bowl in the fridge until ready to use. However, fresh and especially locally grown would be great too!*

1 cup cold apple juice or water
3 Tbsp. bulk gelatin
2 cups apple juice, heated to near boiling
1 packet Pruvit Keto/OS Heart Tart, optional but soooo good!
1 tsp.+ honey or sweetener, optional
1/2+ 16 oz. bag frozen and thawed strawberries, larger ones cut in half

Pour cold juice or water in glass or ceramic bowl. Whisk in gelatin, followed by the Heart Tart ketones, if using. Pour in heated juice, and whisk well one minute, until well dissolved. Taste, and add sweetener if desired. Let sit five minutes, then stir in strawberries. Refrigerate to set.

Variations for Fruit & Juice Jello Recipes:

- Sub the juice of one lime for the Pruvit Heart Tart to add a little tart flavor, then sweeten as needed
- Sub mango or papaya juice for some or all of the apple juice, and sub frozen and thawed mango chunks for the strawberries
- Try any fruit juice + fruit combo that inspires you!

Apple Peach Splash Jello

1 cup cold peach or apricot nectar, apple-peach juice, or plain apple juice
1 Tbsp. glycine, optional
3 Tbsp. bulk gelatin
2 cups apple juice, heated
1 packet Pruvit OS NAT Splash ketones (charged or caffeine-free), optional
1 peach, peeled, pitted, and sliced into small pieces

Pour cold juice into a glass or ceramic bowl. Whisk in glycine, then sprinkle gelatin on top. Whisk well, then add Pruvit Splash packet if using. Whisk in heated apple juice into the gelatin mixture. Let sit for five minutes. Add peach slices. Refrigerate until set.

Apple Pineapple Splash Jello

1 cup cold apple juice or water
3 Tbsp. bulk gelatin
1 Tbsp. powdered glycine
1 packet Pruvit Keto/OS NAT Splash therapeutic ketones
2 cups apple juice, heated
2-3 pineapple rings, torn (from canned, unsweetened) + 2 Tbsp. of the pineapple juice

Pour cold juice or water into a glass or ceramic bowl. Whisk in glycine, then sprinkle gelatin on top. Whisk well, then add Pruvit Splash packet if using. Whisk heated apple juice into the gelatin mixture. Let sit for five minutes. Tear or cut pineapple rings, then stir into the jello mix, along with the pineapple juice. Refrigerate to set.

Cherry Punch Jello

1 cup cold cherry juice, or water
1 Tbsp. powdered glycine, optional
3 Tbsp. bulk gelatin
1 packet Pruvit Keto/OS Maui Punch, optional but really adds a punch!
2 cups apple juice, heated
1/2+ bag frozen and thawed cherries (1-2 cups)

Pour cold juice or water in glass or ceramic bowl. Whisk in glycine, then sprinkle gelatin on top. Whisk well, then add Maui Punch packet if using. Whisk heated juice into the gelatin mixture. Let sit five minutes. Add cherries, then refrigerate to set.

Coconut Jello

2 cups cold coconut milk (I use canned coconut milk)
3 Tbsp. bulk gelatin
1 cup boiled water
Juice of one lime, or 1 packet Pruvit Holy Grail, coconut lime flavored ketones (not always available)
2-3 tsp. honey, coconut sugar, or sweetener of choice
Honey, coconut sugar, and berries or fruit, garnish

Pour cold coconut milk into a glass or ceramic bowl, then vigorously whisk in gelatin, followed by lime or optional Holy Grail ketones, & honey or sugar. Pour boiled water on top, and whisk another minute until gelatin is well dissolved. Let sit five minutes, then refrigerate to set.

To serve, score jello into 6-9 wedges. Place servings into a small bowl, and top with fruit, honey, and coconut sugar as above.

Variations to Coconut Jello Recipe:

- Add 1-2 Tbsp. finely shredded unsweetened coconut
- Add 2 Tbsp. juice from canned pineapple, then serve with pineapple rings, and a drizzle of honey on top

Orange Mango Coconut Jello

1 cup cold orange juice
3 Tbsp. gelatin
1 scoop Pruvit Orange Swirl, optional (also contains whey)
2 cups pure coconut milk (I used canned, not the watered down versions)
1-2+ Tbsp. coconut sugar, or honey (to taste)
1-2 cups thawed frozen mango, cut into smaller pieces, or 1 fresh
Honey & coconut sugar, garnish

Heat 2 cups coconut milk on medium heat until just beginning to steam, but not boil. Separately, add cold juice to a medium bowl. Stir or whisk in the gelatin. It will get a little thick. Add coconut sugar or honey, and Pruvit Orange Swirl if using. (Add a bit more orange juice if needed to dissolve.)

Stir in warmed coconut milk. Let sit about 5 minutes. Add mango, do a quick stir. Refrigerate until firm.

To serve, use a knife to score into 6-9 wedges. Dish out a wedge, then drizzle with honey, and sprinkle coconut sugar on top. Delicious!

Milk Jello ~ aka Low-Fat Panna Cotta

1 cup cold milk &/or water
3 Tbsp. gelatin (Use 3 Tbsp. for stiffer jello, less for less stiff)
2 cups milk, heated (I use whole milk, or 1/2 each whole + 2%)
2 tsp. vanilla
1/4 cup honey or real maple syrup
1-2 tsp. sugar, optional
Honey, coconut sugar, & fresh raspberries, or diced fresh fruit like peaches or papaya, garnish

Heat 2 cups milk until just beginning to steam. Be careful not to scald. Separately, pour cold milk &/or water into a bowl. Sprinkle gelatin on top. Whisk well. Add vanilla, honey, and sugar if using. Once the milk has heated, add to the gelatin mixture. (If you have honey sticking to the measuring cup, pour heated milk into the cup first, then add to the bowl.) Whisk, let sit five minutes, then refrigerate to set. Keeps up to one week.

When serving, score 6-9 sections with a knife. Place 1-2 wedges into a small bowl. Add fresh berries, papaya, or other fruit. Drizzle honey over the top, then sprinkle coconut sugar over the honey. Tastes like pudding or a creme brûlée!

Chocolate Milk Jello Variations:

- Add 2 Tbsp. cocoa powder, 1/2 tsp. ground cinnamon & 1/8 tsp. cardamom or a pinch of nutmeg to the milk while it's warming, then whisk into the cold milk with the gelatin, and remaining ingredients
- For extra ease, add 1 packet Pruvit Swiss Cacao, or Chocolate Swirl instead of the cocoa powder and honey. Taste, and add sweetener as desired

Creamcycle Milk Jello/Low-Fat Panna Cotta Variation

1 cup cold orange juice
3 Tbsp. bulk gelatin
1 scoop Pruvit Orange Swirl Keto OS
2 cups milk, heated
2 Tbsp. honey or 2-3 tsp. sugar

Honey, coconut sugar, & fresh raspberries, papaya, peaches or other fruit, garnish

Heat 2 cups of milk until just beginning to steam. Be careful not to scald. Separately, pour orange juice into a bowl. Sprinkle gelatin on top, and whisk well.

Whisk Pruvit Orange Swirl into warmed milk, then pour into bowl with orange juice and gelatin. Whisk well. Add honey or sugar, then taste a little on a spoon to see if desired sweetness. Let sit five minutes, then refrigerate to set.

To serve, score jello with a knife into 6-9 wedges. Place serving in a small bowl, and top with fresh berries or fruit, a drizzle of honey and sprinkle of coconut sugar, as above.

More Sweet Treats

Poached Pears

2 pears, cut in half and cored
1/2 cup water
1 inch piece of ginger, minced or grated in a ginger grater
Pinch sea salt
About 3/4 tsp. +/- cinnamon

Place pears and water in a small pot. Add minced ginger, or squeeze if grated to get out juice. Sprinkle with cinnamon, and a grind of sea salt. Bring to boil, then turn to medium-low, cover and simmer until pears are soft, about 15-20 minutes. Serve in a bowl with yogurt, ricotta cheese, Mascarpone, or fresh whipped cream.

Alternative preparation methods:

- Place pears in a steamer basket and steam instead of poaching
- Bake in the oven, adding a little apple juice instead of water, and optional butter pats. Bake at 375° until soft.

Rose Hip & Apple Compote ~ *Rose hips are a potent source of bioflavonoids with many great health benefits. Look for bulk rose hips at a local herb or bulk tea shop, or order from Amazon through my links in the Resources chapter at the end.*

4 medium apples (tart, crisp and juicy apples are good)
1/3 cup dried rose hips
1/4 cup raisins
Pinch of sea salt
Water ~ up to 1/2 cup (or use apple cider or juice)

Peel apples. Grate two, and chop the other two. If you don't have a grater, chop them all. In a 4-5 quart heavy-bottom pot, layer ingredients in this order: rose hips, raisins, grated apples, chopped apples, salt, then enough water (or juice) to just cover the bottom of the pot by 1/4-1/2 inch.

Cover, bring to a boil, then reduce heat to low, and simmer 15-20 minutes. If all the apples are chopped, versus grated, simmer for 25-30 minutes. Do not stir while cooking.

Once cooked, stir, then divide among individual serving dishes. It will thicken a bit as it cools. Chill first, or serve warm, topped with yogurt, ricotta cheese, Mascarpone, &/or a drizzle of real maple syrup, honey, or coconut sugar as desired.

Simple Crustless Cheesecake with Cherry Glaze
I adopted this recipe from the Easy Crustless Cheesecake on Cookpad.

2 8 oz. packages of cream cheese, softened
3 eggs
1/4 cup honey
1/4 cup sugar
Zest & juice of 1 lemon
1 tsp. vanilla, optional (skip if you want more lemony flavor)
A buttered round glass pie plate

Preheat oven to 350°.
Whip softened cream cheese in a mixing bowl until soft using a hand blender. Add remaining ingredients, and whip until well combined, free of

lumps. Pour into pie plate. If able, place plate in a bigger roasting pan, and add water about half way up the pie plate. This helps the cheesecake bake more evenly. Bake for about 35 minutes, until a toothpick inserted comes out clean.

Cherry Glaze

1 cup frozen and thawed cherries
Splash of water
1/2 cup cold concord grape juice + 2 tsp. gelatin
1 Tbsp. powdered Swerve, confectioners sugar, or granulated sugar
.5 tbsp. kudzu or arrowroot dissolved in 2 Tbsp. cool water
Pinch of cinnamon, optional

Pour cold juice into a bowl, then add gelatin, and whisk well. Place cherries in a saucepan with splash of water, and begin to simmer on medium heat. Add the grape juice, and let simmer until the cherries begin to soften. Use a fork or potato masher to mash them while simmering in the pot.

In a small dish, mix the kudzu or arrowroot with just enough cool water until dissolved, then add to pot, along with cinnamon if using. Let simmer a few more minutes until thickened. When cheesecake and glaze have cooled, spoon glaze on top, spreading with a knife or spatula. Let chill in the fridge one hour or more before serving.

Notes: You can use a little more gelatin if you don't have any kudzu or arrowroot around. Cornstarch can be used instead of either in a pinch if necessary. Both the gelatin and the kudzu have health benefits. And yes, I love this with blackberries for breakfast!

Coconut Macaroons

4 egg whites
1/4 tsp. cream of tartar
2 & 1/2 cups shredded coconut
1/4 cup coconut flour
1 Tbsp. coconut oil
1/4 cup honey, sugar, or coconut sugar
2 tsp. vanilla
Juice of about 1/4 lemon

Line a big baking sheet with parchment paper. Preheat oven to 300°.

Using a hand mixer, whip egg whites and cream of tartar until stiff peaks begin to form. Blend in sweetener, coconut oil, lemon, and vanilla.

In a separate bowl, combine shredded coconut and coconut flour. Fold in egg white mixture. Use a spoon to scoop up some of the dough to create a cone shape with your hands. They will be about 1-1.5 inches tall (not too big). Place on baking tray, about 1 inch apart. Bake for ~ 40-45 minutes, until light golden brown on the bottom.

Notes: If mixture doesn't hold together well, try wetting your hands, or if needed, add a little more coconut flour.

Chocolate Covered Coconut Macaroon Variation

Place 4 oz. 85-90% dark chocolate cut up in chunks into a small stainless steel or heat proof bowl, and place bowl over a pot half filled with water, on medium heat until chocolate melts.

Turn off heat, and carefully dip maroons into the chocolate, then place on a wax paper lined tray or plate. Let cool, or refrigerate.

6 - CARROT SALADS

A (raw) carrot a day helps keep the excess endotoxins and estrogen at bay!

Carrot Salad Basic Recipe

1 lb. peeled carrots
Juice of 1 orange, 2 limes, or 2 Tbsp. orange juice
1 Tbsp. apple cider vinegar
2 Tbsp. single source XVOO, or Pruvit 1:4:3 MCT oil blend *(Note: Make your own blend: mix 3 parts coconut oil with 4 parts MCT oil together so that the coconut oil remains liquid, and will be a bit less coconut-y flavor.)*
2 tsp. honey
Pinch salt, optional

Shred peeled carrots in a food processor or using a grater, or create shavings with a potato peeler. Place in a glass or ceramic bowl.

Squeeze citrus into a small bowl, and add remaining ingredients. Stir into carrots. Enjoy as is, or try any of the following variations.

Coconut Carrot Salad

1 lb. peeled carrots
2 Tbsp. unsweetened finely shredded coconut
Juice of 1 orange, 2 limes, or 2 Tbsp. orange juice
1 Tbsp. apple cider vinegar

2 Tbsp. XVOO, or 1/2 Packet Pruvit 1:4:3 Virgin Coconut MCT Oil, or make your own blend as described above
2-3 tsp. honey
1/2+ tsp. ground cinnamon, optional
Pinch salt

Shred or shave peeled carrots, and place in a bowl. Stir in shredded coconut. Juice the citrus in a smaller bowl, then stir in the remaining ingredients. Combine with carrots.

Apple Raisin Carrot Salad

Add 1/4 cup raisins, 1/2 peeled and diced apple, and 1 tsp. ground cinnamon to the above **Carrot Salad Basic Recipe**, or the **Coconut Carrot Salad Recipe**. To prevent oxidation of the apple, add before serving.

Apricot Carrot Salad

Omit raisins, and add fresh chopped apricot to either the **Carrot Salad Basic Recipe**, or the **Coconut Carrot Salad Recipe**.

Pineapple Carrot Salad

Make either the **Carrot Salad Basic Recipe**, or the **Coconut Carrot Salad Recipe**, above, using the juice of 2 limes in lieu of the orange juice, then add the following:

3 canned unsweetened pineapple rings, torn into smaller pieces + 2 Tbsp. of the pineapple juice. Additionally add raisins if desired.

Savory Carrot Salad

1 lb. peeled and shredded carrots
Juice of 2 limes
1 Tbsp. apple cider vinegar
2 Tbsp. single source XVOO
1/8-1/4 tsp. salt
1-2 scallions, finely chopped
1 small handful of fresh parsley, basil, or mint, finely chopped
1/8-1/4 tsp. ground cumin
Pinch each of cinnamon & cayenne pepper
Handful of raisins
Drizzle of honey

Combine ingredients in a bowl. Taste test, and add more salt, sweetness (honey/cinnamon), sour (lime/vinegar), savory (cumin), or spice (cayenne) as desired.

7 - VEGGIE SIDES

Enjoy vegetables as desired. Generally speaking, we favor root vegetables over leafy greens and modern cultivated vegetables, especially the cruciferous family which if under cooked, and over consumed can inhibit thyroid function.

Carrot Onion & Hijiki Stir Fry

1+ Tbsp. XVOO or coconut oil
1 small sweet onion, sliced, cut into chunks or half moons
1 stalk celery, sliced on an angle
Pinch of salt
1 inch pc. ginger, minced
2 - 3 carrots, cut diagonally on the bias
2 scallions, cut into 1 inch pieces
About 1/4 cup hijiki, arame, or dulse seaweed* (see below)

*If using hijiki or arame seaweed, soak first to soften. If using dulse, skip soaking, simply cut into small pieces, and add at the end of cooking.

Heat a wok or large pan, then add oil. Once heated, add onion and celery, and let cook 4-5 minutes, undisturbed. Add ginger, and seaweed if using hijiki or arame. Stir fry for a few minutes before adding carrots. Continue stirring and cooking at a medium-high heat for several minutes, until carrots begin to soften. Add scallion, and cook another few minutes.

If using dulse, add, then cover, turn off heat, and let sit a couple minutes.

Variations

- Add 1 tsp. turmeric or sweet yellow curry powder and 1/2 tsp. oregano just before adding carrots
- Add 1/2 cup of bone broth, water, or apple juice after adding carrots, cover, and let simmer on low heat. Again, if using dulse, wait until the end to add
- Add 1 tsp. honey or a pinch of stevia or sweetener at the end of cooking
- Add chopped parsley at the end, or add other vegetables as desired

Pan-Fried Cabbage

Although I do not eat cruciferous veggies as often, this is my fave. Cook cabbage until soft, like noodles! A fun veggie side when in the mood.

1 lg. sweet or yellow onion, sliced
1/2 head of cabbage, sliced horizontally into 1/4 inch wedges in the shape of fettuccine noodles
1 Tbsp. each XVOO + butter, or coconut oil + butter
Salt & white pepper
1 tsp. turmeric or curry powder
1/3 tsp. ground fennel (whole seeds can be ground in a designated coffee grinder)

Heat a deep pan, and add oil + butter. Add onions, and let cook 2-3 minutes before adding cabbage.

Season with salt and pepper and remaining seasonings. Stir to evenly coat the entire mixture. Cover, and let cook on medium-low heat about 10 minutes, until cabbage is soft. Alternatively, add 1/4 cup bone broth before covering with a lid. Also good with a little coconut milk stirred in at the end.

Cucumber Salad

1 cucumber, peeled, deseeded, and chopped
1 fresh tomato, chopped
1/4 red or sweet onion, finely diced
Juice of 1/2+ lemon
2 Tbsp. XVOO
Salt & pepper
Dulse seaweed, rinsed, and cut into small pieces

Combine ingredients in a bowl, and toss gently.

Variations:

- Add chopped sheep, goat, or cow feta cheese
- Add 1/2-1 avocado
- Rinse and soak wakame or alaria seaweed, then sub for the dulse
- Toss Cucumber Salad with canned mackerel, oysters, or crab meat

Roasted Carrots & Parsnips

4+ each carrots & parsnips, peeled

2 Tbsp. XVOO
3 Tbsp. apple cider or juice, or 2 Tbsp. cider vinegar
1 tsp. honey

Choose:
- 1/2 tsp. cinnamon + a pinch each of ground clove & nutmeg
- 1 tsp. dried rosemary + 1/4 tsp. ground sage
- 1 tsp. Italian herb blend or 1/2 tsp. each oregano & basil

Salt and pepper

Preheat oven to 375° and cover a baking sheet with parchment paper.

Cut carrots and parsnips into thirds or quarters, length-wise. Cut each section in half length-wise, then cut each half across on an angle, creating triangular wedge shapes.

Place vegetables and remaining ingredients ~ including whichever herb/seasoning blend you prefer ~ in a large bowl. Toss until well coated. Spread onto baking sheet. Roast for 30-40 minutes. The longer they roast, the sweeter they get!

Roast Winter Squash

2 Kabocha, acorn, or delicata squash
1/4 cup orange juice
3/4 tsp. cinnamon
1/4 cup honey

2 tsp. XVOO or coconut oil or a blend of both
1/4 tsp. each salt & black pepper
Pinch of cayenne pepper

Pre-heat oven to 400° and cover baking sheet with parchment paper.

Cut squash in half, and scoop out seeds. Place open side down on a baking sheet. Bake 45-60 minutes. The outer skin may blacken, and should be soft when pressing.

Combine remaining ingredients in a small bowl. Turn squash right side up. Spoon mixture on top and in center of squash. Use a pastry brush to brush all over if easier. Bake another 10 minutes. Remove from heat, and serve. Ideal as part of a fall/winter holiday meal.

8 - BEVERAGES

For me, a sweet life starts with a great morning beverage!

Orange juice, alone or stir in 1/2 Tbsp. powdered glycine, or 1 Tbsp. gelatin. I sometimes stir in 1/8 tsp. powdered magnesium. *Contrary to popular opinion, orange juice is refreshing and invigorating, especially first thing in the morning, plus it helps eliminate endotoxins from the gut.*

Sparkling Grape Drink

In a glass, combine 2/3 full with Concord grape juice, and 1/3 sparkling water, plain or flavored. Especially good with a Berry flavored water.

Cafe Au Lait

8 oz. milk
1 full tsp. raw, creamy honey
4+ oz. hot brewed coffee

Heat milk, until steaming, but not scalding and pour into large mug. Stir in honey, then add coffee. Stir, and enjoy.

Collagen Coffee

1/4 cup milk, half and half or a blend, or use cold water

1 Tbsp. bulk beef gelatin
12 oz. hot brewed coffee
1+ tsp. honey, or sweetener of choice
1/2 tsp. each MCT oil + coconut oil, optional

Add milk and/or half and half (or water) to mug, and sprinkle gelatin on top. Stir to dissolve. It will be lumpy, nearly like a porridge. If too much so, add more milk. Once combined, add coffee, honey, and optional oil, stir and enjoy.

If motivated, blend in a blender until frothy. If the cold milk cools off the coffee too much, do a quick heat of the milk + coffee in a small saucepan. We often stir gelatin into leftover cool coffee, then heat it.

Coffee with Pruvit Keto Sweet Kreme

Add 1 packet of Pruvit Keto Sweet Kreme to your mug, stir in your coffee, sip, and savor your morning! Quite delicious, and enough of what you need to jump start your morning!

Each packet of Sweet Kreme is 130 calories, and contains 12g of fat (11g saturated), 3g carbohydrate, 2g protein, 5mg vitamin B6, 100mcg B12, 130mg of calcium, 70mg sodium, 40mg potassium, ketones, and collagen derived from Avian sternum and eggshell membrane. It's sweet with a slight taste of cinnamon, and quite delicious!

Rose Hips Tea (*Good source of bioflavonoids and vitamin C*)

4 cups cold filtered water
3 Tbsp. dried rose hips
Honey, stevia, or sugar as desired

Place water and rose hips in a non-metal pot. Simmer on medium heat for about 15 minutes. Strain. Sweeten before cooling, then refrigerate.

I often add a pinch more rose hips, and 2 more cups of water, simmering the second batch a little longer, then add strained tea to the first batch.

Rose hips tea is very refreshing with a little sparkling water.

Variations:

- **Rose Hips & Hibiscus Tea** ~ Use 2 Tbsp. each of rose hips and dried hibiscus flowers, prepared as above, or with any of the following extras
- Add a cinnamon stick
- Add a 2 inch or so piece of dried citrus peel
- Add 1 Tbsp. Chinese chrysanthemum flowers ~ a mellow flavor herbal tea in buds or flowers ~ excellent cooling herb to drink to balance the summer heat, & treat sore throats; also beneficial for the eyes

Roasted Dandelion & Chicory *A nice alternative to coffee, plus dandelion root is great for the liver*

4 cups filtered water
1/8 cup roasted dandelion root
1/8 cup roasted chicory root
1 2-3 inch (aged/dried) citrus peel, optional
Extras: 1 cinnamon stick, 5-6 cardamom pods, pinch of Chinese star anise or fennel seeds, 1 tsp. licorice root, Chinese dang gui herb (angelica root) which helps build the blood, and has a slight licorice taste

Place ingredients in a pot, along with any desired extras. Bring just barely up to a boil, then reduce heat to low and simmer, covered about 10 minutes. Strain, then refill with half the amount of cold water, and a pinch each of fresh herbs, simmer about 20 minutes. Add to first batch. Enjoy as is, or with warmed milk and honey.

Notes:

- When making loose teas, roots can be simmered gently fully or partially covered, however more delicate flowers and stems should just be steeped in hot water for 5+ minutes.
- Citrus peels help break up stagnation. Save citrus peels in a bowl until dry. Store in jars. Add a 2 to 3 inch piece to tea, or look for aged/dried citrus peel in bulk at herb stores or Asian markets.

- Green and black teas contain tannins, and become more bitter the longer they steep. Some people have issues with the strong tannins in teas. Enjoy teas as desired or tolerated. They do provide a small amount of manganese which is beneficial.

6 - RESOURCES

PRODUCTS *I have provided product links in the Kindle version, for informational purposes and to order if interested. You can find recommendations for products on my website at* live-fruitfully.com.

Red Light has many health benefits! Read more:
https://www.fullrangestrength.com/red-light.html
Order a red light here: http://bit.ly/37zdnxS

Bulk Beef Gelatin
I listed a few bulk gelatin alternatives which are a good quality and value, below. Choose what works best for your needs and budget. Products sold as 'collagen' is gelatin that has been hydrolyzed so it dissolves better in hot liquids, but costs more.

NOW Bulk Beef Gelatin - Bulk is best value. Around .67¢ per oz. on average for 4lb.

Zen Principle Beef Gelatin, 3lb.

Knox Unflavored Gelatin 2-pack - https://amzn.to/2NcfbX8

Bulk Supplements Glycine Powder - https://amzn.to/2BnPdsJ

Bulk herbs used in the teas available from Frontier and other companies on Amazon.
VitaminSea Dulse Flakes:

Pruvit Exogenous Flavored Ketones best deal is smart ship which saves 22%, plus they send a free box every fourth month.
Visit: https://tracyminton.pruvitnow.com/products/

Trader Joe's is a good source for sorbate-free dried fruit

Nature's Sunshine is a solid company that has created high quality, bioavailable supplements for several decades. I have a list of my top commonly recommended supplements at: https://www.live-fruitfully.com/natures-sunshine.html. Or visit www.naturessunshine.com and use my referral number 60784000.

We also use **Standard Process,** which produces high quality, whole-foods based herbs they grow, and very absorbable, well formulated supplements. You can find my top recommendations on my website on the Nature's Sunshine tab, with links to purchase on Amazon, or contact us at our Barefoot Acupuncture Clinic if you would like help with preparing a protocol. Read more here: http://www.barefoot-acupuncture.com/functional-nutrition.html.

Swanson Vitamins is an affordable mail order supplier of vitamins and a variety of other products. The Y.S. Eco Bee Farms Raw Honey is an excellent deal. If first time shopping at Swanson's, write this URL in your browser to receive $10 OFF $50: https://www.talkable.com/x/2ThvuB

Costco and Sprouts also have excellent Raw Honey in larger containers for a better value

BOOKS

THE HYPERCARNIVORE DIET, Don Matesz - An excellent, well-referenced book.
NUTRITION AND PHYSICAL DEGENERATION, Weston A. Price
HAIR LIKE A FOX: A BIOENERGETIC VIEW OF PATTERN HAIR LOSS, Danny Roddy
THE CHEROKEE HERBAL, J.T. Garret
CHINESE DIETARY THERAPY, Liu Jilin (main editor)
THE STRONG SPIRIT 10-STEP PLAN, Tracy A. Minton-Matesz - Overcome obstacles to realizing your goals, including weight loss

WEBSITES

Don's website: www.donmatesz.com.
Tracy's website: www.live-fruitfully.com
Our blog: www.thehypercarnivore.com
Ray Peat's website: www.raypeat.com
Danny Roddy's Weblog: www.dannyroddy.com -

Made in the USA
Coppell, TX
23 June 2021